Slow Up

PAMELA ALLARDICE

Slow Up

199 WAYS TO CALM YOUR MIND, RELAX YOUR BODY AND INSPIRE YOUR SPIRIT

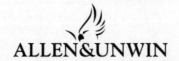

ALLEN&UNWIN

First published in 2006

Allen & Unwin Pty Ltd
83 Alexander Street
Crows Nest NSW 2065
Australia
Phone: (61 2) 8425 0100
Fax: (61 2) 9906 2218
Email: info@allenandunwin.com
Web: www.allenandunwin.com

National Library of Australia
Cataloguing-in-publication entry:
Allardice, Pamela.
Slow up : 199 ways to calm your mind, relax your body and inspire your spirit.

ISBN 1 74114 622 4.

1. Stress management. 2. Relaxation. I. Title.

613

Designed by Nada Backovic
Edited by Foong Ling Kong
Typeset by Prowling Tiger Press
Printed in Australia by McPherson's Printing Group

10 9 8 7 6 5 4 3 2 1

The author and publisher thank Vixen Australia
for the generous loan of the cover outfit.
www.vixenaustralia.com

To Doug, Edward and Randall

Contents

QUICK HELP GUIDE

Do you wish you could start slowing down, quickly?
125, 128, 132, 144, 146, 147, 215, 240

Are you stuck in a rut?
15, 20, 26, 42, 67, 96, 103, 216, 240, 244

Feeling headachey?
85, 20, 180, 244

Do you have trouble getting going in the morning?
8, 10, 182, 191, 209, 221, 223

Have you lost touch with the outside world?
24, 32, 39, 41, 43, 47, 68

Have you forgotten how to enjoy time with your kids?
45, 39, 54, 65, 101

Want to let go of bad habits?
92, 93, 97, 132, 133

Do you need a treat?
22, 62, 65, 75, 83, 218

Are your spirits sagging?
47, 110, 111, 118, 129, 137, 139, 146, 185,

Is work getting you down?
20, 47, 84, 119, 142, 204, 208

Do you feel like you've lost focus?
38, 126, 146, 153, 178

Do you feel irritable and negative?
102, 134, 137, 139, 146, 154, 181, 201, 202

Would you like an energy boost?
167, 171, 174, 176, 177, 191, 193, 195, 198, 223, 228

Does your life feel unbalanced?
140, 142, 151, 172, 177, 186, 187, 153, 195, 215

Do you feel anxious?
157, 170, 182, 226, 237

Are you feeling overwhelmed?
54, 136, 154

Do you feel dull and worn out?
82, 156, 162, 163, 185

Do your feet feel flat?
165, 181, 200

Is your back buckling under the load?
168, 169, 176, 188, 189, 192, 193, 194, 208, 203, 204

Do you need a quick pick-me-up?
11, 79, 180, 202

Is your heart feeling the pressure?
135, 154, 192, 226, 227, 233, 239

Do you get sick too often?
167, 220, 223, 231, 234, 241

HOW DO YOU KNOW
WHEN IT'S TIME TO SLOW UP?

It probably sounds strange to say that I got the idea for this book after getting eleven stitches in my chin. I had been given the go-ahead by my publisher to start writing, and I had entered that agonising period known as 'getting into the book'. I was cranky, I hated my family and I couldn't sleep. I tried writing in the kitchen, the lounge room, the bedroom and on the back verandah – all with the same result: nothing. Zip.

I moped, I slammed doors, and then I called my mother.

'Just calm down and relax, dear,' she said. 'Do something else to take your mind off it, and the ideas will come.'

Calm down and relax? How could I, when I had so much to do? And when I was constantly stopping whatever I was trying to do – 'Try and remember where you put the big screwdriver', 'Read the directions and see if it works on slugs as well', 'Give me that recipe for poppyseed cake', 'Is it OK if the whole football team comes here for dinner, and then they all sleep over?' As I was brooding, a siren-like wail came from Randall's room.

'Mum, Edward's wrecking my project. Make him stop!' Grimly, I went upstairs to act as referee to my two disagreeable sons (mere gesture), only to trip and fall all the way down, rearranging my jaw and two teeth, and splitting my chin to the bone.

Six hours later I was lying in bed feeling very sorry for myself. The boys slid into the room.

'Do you want to see what I made?'

'Do you feel like getting up now?'

No, I did not.

Doug called Mum, who came on the next bus, bringing peace, commonsense and cups of strong, sweet tea.

'I am so depressed,' I said tearfully. 'I have so much to do, and I'm worried about the kids and Doug, and now this.'

'I don't know why you would worry about the boys and Doug. Running the house will be a good experience for them. Get a good night's sleep and put it all out of your mind. Having this happen is probably a blessing in disguise, because it means you're forced to have a rest,' she said.

As I lay there listening to the sounds of the boys valiantly 'keeping quiet for Mum' (they kept it down to hissed insults, two slaps and seven phone calls) I realised that all over the world there are other exhausted women who, under similar circumstances, are definitely not relaxing. Like me, they want more balance in their lives. I also realised that dramatic solutions – like moving to an island or signing up for a silent Buddhist retreat – weren't going to work because I actually quite liked my life the way it was; I just needed to manage stress better and be more mindful of the things that really mattered.

'Don't compromise yourself,' said Janis Joplin. 'You're all you've got.'

Short of taking a two-week holiday to a desert island, you can refresh your spirit, focus your mind, and get some much-needed perspective. That much, I did learn. Here are 199 of the tips, ideas, and techniques that have helped me muddle through. Think of them not just as first-aid for when you're tired, but as small steps towards a whole strategy for creating long-term harmony and vitality in your life, and staying sane in an insane world. It's never too late to take the first step – even if it does take eleven stitches to make you do it.

'Study nature, love nature, stay close to nature. It will never fail you.'

FRANK LLOYD WRIGHT

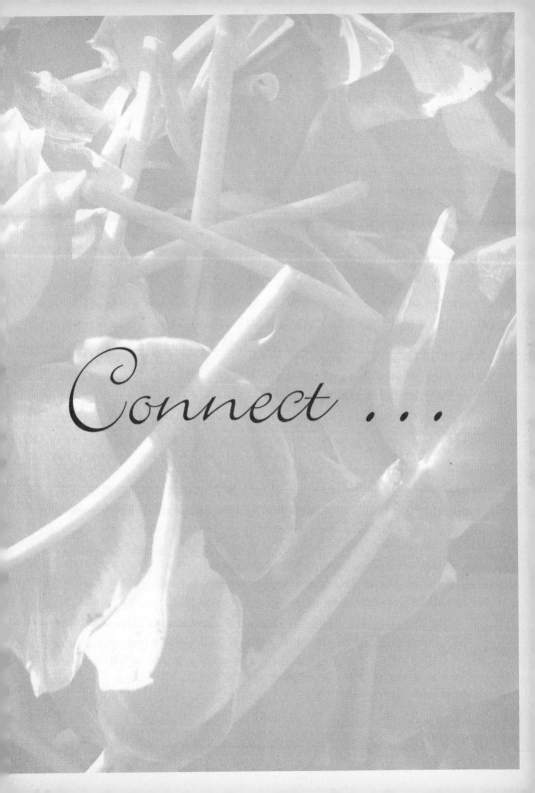

Connect . . .

Staying connected to the natural world will relax your body, free your mind, and restore a sense of balance and perspective. The earth's bounty is infinitely healing and calming. Spending time in nature soothes an over-excited nervous system, and it remains the one universal cure for stress and despair. Despite being surrounded by privation and unimaginable horror and despair, Anne Frank was able to write, 'The best remedy for those who are afraid, lonely or unhappy is to go outside, somewhere they can be quiet, alone with the heavens, nature, and God. Because only then does one feel that all is as it should be and that God wishes people happy, amidst the simple beauty of Nature.'

Get out of bed, go outside and take a breath of fresh air. Soak up the morning's beauty before everyone else wakes up. Admire the washed-clean bright blue of the sky after it's rained, listen to the magpies' liquid call, touch the graceful strip of bark peeling from a gum tree. Feel the sun on your face, and let the wind lift your hair and play with it. Go barefoot whenever you can. Kick off your shoes and let yourself feel the grass or sand beneath your feet. A symbol of connection with the earth and our personal freedom, it's also one of the quickest of all ways to slow down, recharge your spirit and find balance in your life.

Can't get outside? Use your imagination. As Albert Einstein said, 'Logic will get you from A to B. But imagination will take you everywhere.' It doesn't matter if you're up to your elbows in soapsuds at the kitchen sink, or studying late at night, you can still close your eyes, take a deep breath, and picture yourself walking along a beach at twilight, diving beneath a wave and tasting the salt water, or sitting on a moss-covered rock and dangling your fingers in the icy-cold water of a mountain stream.

By creating a meaningful connection with something – whether it's nature, family, a partner, work or a complete stranger – you begin to believe in something larger than yourself. Shifting your attention from (un)civilisation to the beauty of the natural world makes you feel more fully alive; it also means that you begin to acknowledge your place in the world, to see the sense of it all. Developing any kind of real passion and authentic purpose will do the trick, too. Go where you're needed: volunteer for a homeless shelter or a political organisation. No one has really said it better since William Shakespeare wrote, 'The quality of mercy is not strained; it is twice blessed; it blesseth him that gives and him that takes.' In other words, if you give to another person and help enrich their life in some way, you are also giving yourself the opportunity to grow and to connect with the world in a meaningful way. Help something to grow, whether it's a child, an animal or a tree. Have real conversations with real people, not machines, wherever you can. Be a person who lifts people up, not someone who brings them down.

Consider the small, tenacious cluster of leaves that somehow manages to grow out of rusty guttering on a building in the middle of the city, or the tender, apple-green spikes that stubbornly poke out of the charred earth hours after a fire has destroyed everything in its path. No matter how stressed your day is, or how difficult it is to see a way forward, you can find solace, inspiration and courage in Nature's resilience and determination.

1. WAKE UP GENTLY

Your emotions and your health are intimately linked. However, finding a few minutes to be alone and quiet every day so that you can try to process your thoughts can often seem impossible. The realities of modern life distract you with their never-ending mental chatter, so you wake up thinking about what you have to do by the end of the day, what you should have done yesterday, or that tough project you've got to tackle next week – anything but what is happening to you right this minute.

Quiet time helps cut through all this noise to help you find out what's really important, what really matters. You may think you don't have the time, but think of it this way: you have exactly the same amount of time in your day as the wisest, calmest and most successful people in the world. It's all about how you spend that time.

Start by taking 5 minutes to meditate first thing each morning. Make it a priority. Just those few minutes will make an enormous difference to how you feel, look, sleep and think. Set your alarm for ten minutes earlier than your usual wake-up time, then, instead of getting up, meditate for 5 to 10 minutes. This is a perfect time to practise, as there are minimal distractions; it will soon become a pleasant routine that connects you to your day's rhythms, like brushing your teeth.

◆ When the alarm goes, hit the snooze button and allow your eyes to gently close. Focus on your breath. Stopping your attention from flying off in all directions is not easy, but with practice you'll find it is a reliable way to create calm, focus your thoughts, and collect your energies, which is especially beneficial just as you're getting out of bed. Take a long, deep breath and imagine it gathering up all your concerns, thoughts and activities. Hold for a count of 5, then exhale.

◆ Continue to breathe slowly and evenly, in for a count of 5, then out for a count of 5. With practice, the pause between each in and out breath will lengthen. Get used to how it feels. Acknowledge all your different thoughts and visualise them becoming less confused, and settling into place with the rise and fall of your breath. Notice how the breath moves all the way through you – filling first your nostrils, then your throat, your chest and belly – and how it increasingly energises and sustains you. Your breath is the source of your power – if you feel yourself being distracted by a particular thought or problem, just return your focus to the movement of your breath.

◆ Continue until the alarm sounds.

Waking to this gentle meditation helps you feel connected, calm and more balanced in two ways. First, it counters your body's tendency to produce the stress chemicals adrenalin and cortisol, which build up in your body, making you tired, irritable and less efficient. Adrenalin and cortisol also compromise your body's ability to fight germs.

Secondly, when you create these few minutes of quiet time each day, something amazing happens: you begin to hear your inner voice. The playwright Goethe said, 'The hardest thing to see is what is right in front of your eyes.' It is only when you are very quiet and still and can distance yourself from the distractions of the day that you get clear answers to the big questions that are right in front of you, such as 'What makes me happy?' and 'Who do I really want to be in my life?'

In time, you may find that you would love to start a herb nursery, or you discover a desire to try wood-turning, or realise that you actually don't want to host the Christmas lunch this year. Author Mark Twain wrote that, 'The worst loneliness is not to know yourself.' Those 5 minutes in the early morning each day will centre you, and reconnect you with your inner voice. Be true to it, and let it guide you on the big and little decisions each day.

2. SEE THE LIGHT

According to the ancient Indian healing tradition, Ayurveda, if you are living a life that is disconnected from natural rhythms – if you are under stress, eating and sleeping poorly, and not taking time to nurture your spirit with meditation and quiet contemplation – then your vital energy, which is known as prana, will be compromised.

Constant exposure to unnatural light sources such as fluorescent lighting in offices is thought to drain energy, have a negative effect on mood, and worsen stress-related ailments such as insomnia. Natural light, on the other hand, has a balancing, restorative effect on emotions and your body's individual rhythms.

A simple way to boost prana – and to feel stronger, less stressed and more focused – is to let yourself be woken by natural light as often as you can. The rays of the rising sun act as a natural trigger to your mind and body, gently shifting you from a dreaming state to a waking one, and then gradually raising your body temperature and charging up your hormones.

Aim to be in bed by 10 p.m. at least three nights a week, and leave your blinds open so that you wake up with the sun. You will feel more relaxed and refreshed, and also more in tune with the day.

3. TAKE A CITRUS SHOWER

Soaking in a tub full of hot, scented water has its benefits, but on busy days, the process of filling that tub and soaking for twenty minutes can seem daunting. On even the most frantic morning, you can turn a two-minute shower into a haven of peace and an opportunity to indulge your senses.

Sprinkle one or two drops of lemon essential oil on the floor of the shower recess. Lemon oil is definitely a blues pick-me-upper. When you inhale the fresh, bracing, head-clearing scent, its properties go beyond the blood–brain barrier, helping to produce an uplifting effect on your mood. One study has even found that depressed patients who were instructed to inhale lemon oil each morning needed fewer antidepressant drugs than those who did not – and some were able to get off their medication altogether. Start your day feeling purposeful and focused with this skin-tingling treatment.

◆ Sprinkle 5 drops of lemon essential oil into a washbasin filled with warm water. Dip a clean face-washer into the water, wring it out, and proceed to briskly massage your body with it, using small firm circles. Start at your feet and move upwards, always moving towards your heart, which helps to stimulate your circulation.

◆ Sprinkle another 5 drops of lemon essential oil on the floor of the shower recess. Run a warm shower (if you make it too hot, you will feel lethargic afterwards, rather than invigorated) and step in. Steam from the warm water helps disperse the oil and spread the aromatherapy benefits without any extra effort on your part.

◆ Finish with a short blast of cold water at the end of your shower for a dynamic wake-up. Make sure you let the water play on the nape of your neck and chest for a super-stimulating effect. Not only does this help shake off whatever grogginess the warm water may have caused, but it also closes your pores, which protects your immune system. When you get out of a steaming-hot shower, all of your pores are left wide open, which means that all the heat is allowed to leave your body.

◆ Towel off, and resolve to keep that fresh, focused feeling with you all day.

4. GREET THE DAY

The Apache Native Americans have a strong spiritual tradition based on their belief that every action, word and thought is an opportunity to connect with the Great Circle of Life. In their culture, meditation does not mean turning inwards for contemplation and self-examination and closing down to stillness and absence of thought. It means opening yourself up to the earth's energies, feeling them flow through you and fill you up, while listening to what the Universe is telling you. They call these signals from nature 'signposts'.

This daily breathing and meditation practice is designed to align you with the unique essence of each day. Live in the day: do not look backwards to the day before or forwards to the day yet to come. By allowing your spirit to flow out into nature, and welcoming the messages, impressions, feelings and energies back into you via your breath, you will start your day feeling centred and peaceful.

◆ **Create a sacred space** This can be inside or outside your home. It can be as basic as a favourite window with a view that you like, or a plant or painting that always gives you pleasure when you look at it. It should be a spot where you feel safe and comfortable, where you can lower your guard and just be yourself.

◆ **Breathe in a circle** Stand in your sacred space. Imagine that you are at the centre of a large wheel, with four spokes radiating out from your feet. These are the four points of the compass. Breathe in deeply, moving both arms inwards in a slow, circular, scooping motion, as if you were giving someone a warm, welcoming hug. Then breathe out and release your arms, opening your chest and closing your eyes. Do this four times, once for north, east, south and west.

◆ **Welcome the day** Feel the different energies flowing in from the four points of the compass you have just addressed. Be ready to go wherever the day wants to take you.

5. WEAR A FLOWER

Before she set out to walk to the station every day, my grandmother would pick a tiny posy of flowers or even just a sprig of rosemary and pin it to her hat or thread it through the brooch on her jacket lapel.

My mother kept the tradition going when I went to school, giving me a flower every morning as I went out the door, to hold or to pin to my shirt. On leaving the house, I still always take a flower – I might tuck it into a buttonhole, leave it on my desk at work, or maybe I'll just put it on the dashboard of the car. One sunny afternoon last summer, I even twined ivy and honeysuckle and nasturtiums into a circle and made a flower crown for a small friend.

'That's not a real crown!' scoffed her brother.

'Yes, it is!' she said. And she wore it for most of the day, skipping through the bush, at one with nature, a fairy princess crowned with rubies and emeralds.

Wearing a flower or carrying the smallest piece of greenery with you during the course of your day is a link with home and with nature. It's also a way of connecting with the pagan child inside you. 'One touch of nature makes the whole world your kin,' wrote William Shakespeare. Don't wait for an invitation to a formal event or dinner to pin a flower to your shirt, or to tuck one behind your ear. Do it today.

6. PLANT A TREE

In earlier, more superstitious times, a tree-planting ceremony was often used to mark the birth of a child. By association, it was thought that the child's future and fortune would be reflected in the tree's. If the tree thrived, so would the child, but if it became ill, it was a warning that something bad might befall the child.

Even if you have only a small garden, you can plant a suitable tree. Ask a nursery for advice on varieties that do not grow more than a certain height, such as Japanese tallow trees or magnolias. Even if you have no yard at all, most councils have tree-planting programs, and you can participate by planting a tree elsewhere, perhaps naming it for yourself or a loved one if you wish. If possible, plant your tree where you will be best able to admire it from the house – from the kitchen window, perhaps, or near the front gate so it greets you each day. Choose a deciduous tree so you can be reminded of the natural cycle of the seasons, and enjoy autumn colours and anticipate bud-burst each spring.

Make your tree-planting ceremony one where you can make a meaningful connection with nature. As you dig the hole for the sapling and before you smooth the soil back around its base, take a few moments to hold the soil in your hands. Shut your eyes and inhale the dark, rich, earthy smell. Crumble it between your thumb and fingers and let it dribble back on the ground. Feel the ancient energy and acknowledge the deep, soothing rhythms of life.

7. TRY A YIN–YANG MEDITATION

The power of mental visualisation can give you a much-needed mental break and help restore your spirit and heighten your senses, even if you only have five minutes to spare. This meditation aims to balance your energies, and to help you become more conscious of the natural world around you and feel more connected to it.

◆ Sit with your back straight, feet flat on the ground. Imagine that the power of the earth is flowing up through the soles of your feet, like water from an underwater spring. This is *yin*, or feminine, energy. Feel the *yin* cooling your temper and steadying your resolve, giving you strength of purpose and control. Breathe in and imagine that you are drawing in more *yin*, and that it is refreshing you as it flows up your spine and neck, then out the top of your head before flowing down the outside of your body, and washing you clean.

◆ Now, visualise the sun overhead, and feel its warm rays falling on the top of your head. The sun represents *yang*, or masculine, energy. Imagine the rays penetrating the top of your head and beaming all the way to the base of your spine, parallel to the gushing cool, clear *yin* energy which continues to flow upwards. Hold this image for several moments: imagine *yin* flowing in and up as you inhale, and *yang* flowing down and out as you exhale.

◆ When the two energy flows are moving in parallel, in perfect balance and harmony, open your eyes and you will feel energised and refreshed.

8. FLOWER POWER

Some plants seem to act as child-magnets, drawing kids to them again and again. Even the tiniest flower can seem like a miracle to a child: consider the personality of a pansy's 'face' or the texture of a woolly lamb's ear.

Of course, every child knows how to tell the time, dandelion style: you blow as hard as you can, then you count the number of puffs left that it takes to blow away the remaining 'clock' or seeds. Next time you see one take a minute to blow out the clock, if there is one. In that moment, you will have kept faith with your own childhood self, as well as connecting with those countless boys and girls who, for centuries, have picked dandelion clocks, closed their eyes and blown. According to tradition, each of the tiny, feathery seeds on a dandelion clock has the power to sail secret messages on the wings of the wind. Perhaps this childlike chill-out technique will blow your hassles away, just for a moment.

And who doesn't remember 'He loves me, he loves me not …'? Somehow – through the centuries and over whole continents, and generally without the benefit of books – gentle, playful traditions have been passed down from generation to generation. How else to explain how the simple, repetitive steps involving making a daisy chain – or a clover chain, if there are no daisies handy – is known by children the world over? Sitting in a park or garden and idly piecing together a daisy chain, with the sun on your hair, you will feel your shoulders relax and your breathing become slower and calmer as your chain lengthens. Relax – simple pleasures are life's treasures.

Daisy Chain

clump of daisies or clover patch

◆ Pick daisies or clover with stems of at least 4 cm (1½ in) long.

◆ Use the very tip of your thumbnail or a tiny point of a nail file or butter knife to make a narrow slit towards the end of the first stem. Make sure you do not cut all the way through to the bottom of the stem.

◆ Slip the second daisy through so that the head fits snugly over the slit. Make a slit in this second stem, thread the third flower and pull it gently into place, and so on.

9. KEEP A GOLDFISH

It's no accident that the dentist usually has an aquarium in the waiting room. Watching fish drift leisurely past in their cool world of floating weed and spiralling bubbles makes you feel calm, relaxed and unhurried.

Set up an aquarium at home, or keep a little fish bowl near your desk. Every so often, just gaze at it and you will find that something quite remarkable happens – you return to those leisurely days of childhood when, fascinated, you pressed your nose against the cold glass of a fish tank at the pet store or the zoo, and watched as the fish nosed over to the glass to watch you. You can buy fish and aquarium kits with filters and pumps from a specialist supplier. Or, it's quite easy to make your own.

Goldfish Tank

> a large glass bowl
> gravel or pebbles
> greenery
> pH salts, from a pet supplies store
> goldfish

◆ Fill the bowl two-thirds full with hot water from the tap, then pour the hot water into another container and leave overnight. This will get rid of some of the chlorine present in tap water.

◆ Wash and dry the bowl and rinse the gravel or pebbles thoroughly. Put the gravel in the bottom of the bowl and plant the greenery, securing the roots in place with a few larger pebbles. Carefully pour in the reserved water. Add the pH salts according to the manufacturer's instructions.

◆ Pop the fish in and feed it with a few flakes of fish food. Change some of the water regularly, using a cup to scoop it up and pour it away, then top up with fresh water, as above. If you get more than one fish, you will need to invest in a pump and filter as the extra fish will need more space and oxygen.

10. START A WORM FARM

When the boys were small, they wanted a worm farm. I was apprehensive, anticipating that I would be the one who had to look after it. Well, I did end up being the mother of thousands but I didn't mind. The most surprising benefit, though, was the enormous satisfaction that I gained from this simple project. Every evening, when I stepped outside and tipped the leftover kitchen scraps under the worm farm lid, I knew that these useful, industrious creatures were quietly working away while I slept, making rich, thick soil for my plants. Keeping worms makes you think about the earth, and how it nourishes you, and how it responds so enthusiastically to even the smallest amount of care and appreciation. You feel a connection with the many generations of humans who have worked with the earth, and you begin to understand why our ancestors saw it as a mother goddess, and worshipped it.

Worm Farm

> large container (the foam cartons used to pack fruit and veg are ideal)
> bedding material, e.g. mixture of peat moss, shredded paper, leaf mould, straw or grass clippings
> soil
> compost
> food, e.g. kitchen scraps
> earthworms
> shadecloth or hessian

◆ Half-fill the container with the bedding material and moisten slightly. Add a thin layer of soil, then a layer of compost, then spread a bit more soil on top.

◆ Tuck a bit of food for the worms just beneath the surface, scratching the soil over it to cover lightly. Put the worms on top of the soil over the buried food – they will soon wriggle downwards to escape the light.

◆ Cover the box loosely with the hessian or shadecloth to provide some shelter and reduce moisture loss.

◆ Sprinkle the soil with water every couple of days. Don't make it too wet as this will foul the soil and kill the worms.

11. WEAR NATURAL FIBRES

Every mother knows that swaddling babies in soft fabric makes them feel settled and secure, and encourages deep, restful sleep. Use the same approach when dressing yourself, opting wherever possible for light, luxurious natural fabrics, like cashmere and linen.

Dress for comfort and grace, not fashion: no sharp shoulders, tight cuffs or uncomfortable high heels. Tight clothes can make you hyperventilate (breathe too fast), add years to your looks, as well as raise your blood pressure. Choose clothes that make you feel calm and connected to your body: floaty skirts that let the warm air kiss your skin, open-collared shirts that let you breathe and turn your head, flat or low-heeled shoes that let you run and walk briskly whenever you choose. Treat yourself to the sensuous pleasures of a delicate silk camisole, a sheer cotton lawn shirt, a treasured angora jumper that you can nestle into. They will delight your senses and help you feel at ease.

Our fundamental motive for getting dressed is actually not for warmth or protection – it is to decorate ourselves and to send messages to the world about who we are. Consider the scarf, which must be one of the oldest forms of clothing – people were wrapping lengths of woven material around their bodies long before anyone figured out how to use a needle and thread, or to sew a seam. A scarf is like a favourite piece of jewellery: the more you wear it, the more it feels like a part of who you are. No buttons, no pulling or tugging, no lacing or belting. Opt for natural fabrics, such as silk chiffon, wool or alpaca … wrap it softly around your throat, knot it around your head, sweep it over your shoulder or thread it through the loops of your jeans. Grace yourself with a flattering fusion of colour and texture.

12. MOVE THROUGH A MIST

Fragrance-heavy air fresheners may mask unpleasant odours from pets, cooking and smoke, but the chemical ingredients can irritate eyes, skin and throat, and make you feel agitated and unsettled. More worryingly, air fresheners and aerosols contribute to a complex build-up of chemicals and volatile organic compounds in the home – researchers have found that some commercial air fresheners and aerosols are associated with an increased risk of ear-aches in children and headaches in adults.

Create a relaxing mood by changing the atmosphere at home or work – literally. Use an aromatherapy burner to vaporise essential oils, or fill a clean spray bottle with 100 ml water, add 4–6 drops of essential oil(s) of your choice, shake well, and use to mist your room, your car seat or your desk. Choose from the following.

◆ **Basil** To focus your mind and boost concentration.

◆ **Lavender** To calm and soothe.

◆ **Clove** To warm and comfort.

◆ **Ylang-ylang** To ground the senses.

◆ **Chamomile** To alleviate stress-related headaches and jitteriness.

13. BATHE BY CANDLELIGHT

While getting clean is, in one sense, utilitarian, bathing also happens to be one of the best (and easiest) things you can do to balance your psyche and restore your sanity ... especially if you add a little atmosphere by burning natural vegetable wax or beeswax candles.

When you take a bath in a room lit by harsh electric bulbs, you remain firmly tethered to the stresses of your working day. Dimming the lights with an automatic dimmer switch can improve the mood, but it doesn't come close to the soothing ambience created by lighting a candle – several is even better – and creating a haven of natural calm and intimacy.

Candlelight takes us back to a simpler, slower-paced time, when humans naturally stopped work when the sun set, instead of trying to squeeze more activities into the night-time hours. Float in the water and gaze at the patterns thrown on the walls by the candlelight. Focus on one flame and draw the idea of the light deep into your mind, putting all other thoughts aside. Watch the soft light play on the water around your body; imagine you've captured the moonlight in your bath. Let the warm, scented water slow your body and brain down.

Lighting candles turns a simple bath into your very own sanctuary. Savour the moment of doing. Absolutely. Nothing.

14. HAVE A CHOCOLATE FACIAL

Your sensuality is an undeniable part of who you are. Contrary to what is depicted in movies, books or advertisements, sensuality is not necessarily about having a beautiful body or even having mind-blowing sex. It is how you live your life, how you connect with others and with yourself that determines what sort of physical energy you put out.

When you are out of touch with your senses, everything else will also be out of balance. Do something today that makes you comfortably aware of your more sensual self. Massage your toes, try a new perfume or feed your skin with this indulgent do-it-yourself chocolate facial. It's a luscious treat for your skin and your sense of smell, and is suitable for all skin types. Cocoa is a source of antioxidants, which have a toning effect, the honey has humectant properties (meaning it helps your skin retain moisture) while the yoghurt adds lactic acid which helps dissolve dead skin cells and refine skin texture.

CHOCOLATE FACIAL

> ¼ cup cocoa powder
> 2 tablespoons honey
> 4 tablespoons natural plain yoghurt
> 1 vitamin E capsule
> rice flour

◆ Combine the first three ingredients to form a sloppy paste.

◆ Snip the end off the vitamin E capsule and squeeze the contents into the mixture. Stir well.

◆ Add enough rice flour to form a smooth, firm, workable texture. Smooth over face and neck, avoiding the eye area and lips. Lie down for 15 minutes. Rinse off with warm water and pat dry.

15. GROW FRESH SPROUTS

According to practitioners of traditional Chinese medicine eating dead food will contribute to dead chi, or stagnant life force, in your body. Eating live, fresh foods, on the other hand, supports the flow of natural life energy.

Despite learning the dry science of it in school, the germination of the smallest plant is still a miracle. Give a little water and light to a tiny, tough seed and – incredibly – it turns into something that can nourish your body as well as your soul. And besides contributing a cheery touch of green to your kitchen windowsill, adding snipped fresh sprouts to sandwiches and salads is one of the quickest and easiest ways to tip the nutrition scales in your favour.

Sprouts are a good source of vitamins A and C and chlorophyll, along with trace elements, minerals and enzymes that are easily lost during cooking and storage.

Buy a seed sprouter, or just use this old-fashioned jar-and-pantyhose method – it will work just as well now as it did in primary school.

SEED SPROUTER

> a wide-mouthed glass jar
> seeds, e.g. alfalfa, mung bean, radish
> piece of pantyhose
> rubber band

◆ Rinse out the jar thoroughly. Put the seeds in the bottom of the jar and cover with water. Cap the jar with the piece of pantyhose and secure to the neck with a rubber band. Leave for 10 minutes, then upend the jar to strain out the water. Shake the jar so that the seeds are evenly distributed along the bottom, not clumped together.

◆ Lay the jar on its side in a warm, light place (but not in direct sunlight).

◆ Repeat the watering and shaking process each morning until the seeds sprout.

16. LIVE IN THE SEASON

Our ancestors revered the life-giving power of the sun and the rain for good reason – they knew that, without them, crops would fail and they would die. In today's artificially lit and air-conditioned world, it is easy to go for days at a time without seeing the sky or the sun. This disconnection from nature is unhealthy for both mind and body. To find balance in our lives, we need to step outside more often, and be more conscious of the seasons and the weather. Living in harmony with the seasons and adopting the pace of nature teaches you patience.

Lord Byron wrote movingly of 'the pleasure in the pathless woods, the rapture on the lonely shore'. However, you don't have to go 'out there' in the wilderness or wait for a perfect summer's day or for the wind to die down before you venture forth.

Living in the season means embracing the elements that are on offer – whether your day has brought you rain, wind, sunshine or all three. It means buying and eating food in season – sipping hot soup in winter, cool drinks in summer – and becoming more fully aware of the world around you. As the naturalist Henry David Thoreau said, 'Live each season as it passes: breathe the air, drink the drink, taste the fruit.' Nature is right here, in and around you, wherever you happen to be – whether you're hanging out the washing, working in an office block or flying overhead.

Go outside, close your eyes and hold your face up to the sun for a few moments. Feel the sun's life-giving rays playing on your skin. Let its warmth soothe your spirit. Feel the renewal. Think of how this burning star has given life to the earth and to you, and to thousands of living beings who have gone before you. Feel the warmth entering your mind, illuminating your thoughts. Cast away your petty worries and concerns as you sense the ancient power of the earth's rhythms.

17. GAZE INTO A FIRE

As a child, I remember sitting on the hearth rug at my grandparents' home as the first fire of autumn was lit. I loved to hear the crackle and snap as the logs embraced the flame, and the marvellous head-clearing scent of eucalyptus twigs, pine cones and soft wood smoke would fill the room. The shelves full of books and journals all wore that faint, sweet scent of wood smoke. Nanna would sit in her rocking chair and crochet, while Pa would sit in his velveteen club chair with the frayed armrests and read or do crosswords. I would lie on my stomach, maybe drawing but mostly staring into the fire, then dozing off and having to be carried to bed by Pa. It is one of my most treasured memories.

Why is looking into a fire such a profoundly calming and inspirational experience? Perhaps it's because fire stirs our simpler, more primal selves – the flames dart upwards and throw out heat to our faces and hands just as they did in our ancestors' days. Modern society divorces us from daily contact with nature, and even human interactions are becoming ever more remote, more virtual. People are so out of touch with ancient, powerful elements – fire, wood and smoke – that they need to stop and just sit together. Gazing into a fire makes us feel contemplative and relaxed, inspired and awed by the power of nature at the same time.

In the cooler months take a few minutes to light a fire, if you have one. Sit back and watch as the flames catch. Feel the heat on your face and watch the smoke and sparks twirl up the chimney, drawing your thoughts and dreams upwards, to the sky and the heavens.

18. GO ON A MENTAL JOURNEY

A simple and effective relaxation technique, guided visualisation is, basically, conscious daydreaming.

Your imagination is a powerful ally in your quest to create a more balanced and connected life. Just as it can rev your body up into a panicked 'fight-or-flight' response by merely thinking about a stressful situation or problem, it can also counter negativity and anxiety, and help you wind down and become calmer by thinking about something peaceful and beautiful. As poet John Milton said, 'The mind is its own place: in itself it can make a heaven of hell, and a hell out of heaven.'

Use this guided meditation to help you become stronger and more centred, more in control and relaxed. By creating scenarios in your mind in which you react the way you would like to react, you build confidence when faced with challenges and conflict, and you begin to live the life you've imagined. The more you practise, the more vivid the images in your mental journey will become, and the time it takes you to fall into a state of deep relaxation will become shorter.

◆ Choose a quiet place where you are unlikely to be disturbed for a little while. Close your eyes and take a few deep breaths.

◆ Cup your palms over your eyes and visualise your 'third eye'. According to yogic tradition, this is the spot in the centre of your forehead that governs intuition, spiritual insight and imagination.

◆ Envisage a resplendent life force – perhaps a beautiful sparkling waterfall, with great plumes of spray rushing up in the air. Visualise yourself stepping towards the waterfall. You can hear the splashing water, feel the cool mist on your cheeks. Appreciate the beautiful deep blue of the water, the dark green ferns around its base, the smooth glistening dark rocks covered with soft, damp moss. Slowly and carefully put yourself in the picture.

◆ Run your fingers in the water beside you as you step towards the waterfall, feel how the top level seems effervescent and full of movement, and how deeper down below the surface the water becomes still and cool. See yourself standing beneath the waterfall, and imagine the water as a force running through your body, flowing through you, washing away your negativity and tiredness as it sinks away into the earth at your feet. Be aware of how completely relaxed and refreshed you are.

◆ If any negative mind-chatter begins to creep in, simply stop and begin again at whichever point of your mental journey that feels comfortable. When you are ready, take your hands from your eyes and place them in your lap. Say, 'I will see clearly and make calm, intelligent decisions for the rest of the day.' Stamp your feet and open your eyes to re-establish contact with the everyday world.

19. INSTALL A WATER FEATURE

Water has long featured in stories and rituals of renewal and healing, and natural springs and waterfalls are often venerated as holy places. The sound of water moving – murmuring, gurgling and splashing – puts you at ease and soothes your soul, plus it catches changing reflections of light and muffles sounds.

Still water also produces a feeling of serenity, and the smallest pond or even a dish of water in a courtyard will create a cool, calm, private atmosphere where you can connect with yourself and with nature.

Even if you have no garden, the tranquil effect of water need never be excluded through lack of space – a courtyard, a balcony, even a hallway, all are suitable locations for a water feature. Nor does it have to be expensive – I once made a water feature out of a discarded laundry tub and a second-hand submersible electric pump. Small readymade kits for wall-fixed fountains or simple spout-and-trough features can be assembled and bolted to an existing internal or external wall in less than an hour, creating an oasis for meditation and contemplation.

Every so often, float a single flower, a handful of petals or one or two floating candles on the surface of your water garden. As you do so, still your mind and think for a moment or two about how the sound of the water pacifies you, and how the cool moisture helps freshen the air you breathe. Dip your fingers into the water as you pass and feel the moisture cool and evaporate on your skin as you move.

20. LIVE IN REAL TIME

The writer H.G. Wells said, 'We must not allow the clock and the calendar to blind us to the fact that each moment of life is a miracle and mystery.' Nothing increases a sense of panic and frustration more than clock-watching, and yet – courtesy of wristwatches, TV, radio, mobile phones, laptops, Palm Pilots and car clocks – we are surrounded by reminders of how little time we have. Reduce time-induced stress by minimising technological monitoring, tuning in-to natural rhythms and setting more realistic goals of how long it takes to perform a particular task. Here are some strategies that may help.

◆ **Play the 'double time' game** Use a stopwatch to time your next lunch-time walk, the dash around the fruit market, dinner with the kids. Then, next time you do that same activity, leave the stopwatch, the wristwatch and the CD-radio at home, and deliberately plan to take twice as long as you did before. Notice how a rushed chore becomes a more measured, calming activity.

◆ **Cut down on clocks** Tour your home and office and take an inventory of the clocks on display. Don't forget to count the digital display in your car or on your mobile phone. Chances are you are prompted by at least ten daily reminders of how quickly time is escaping from your grasp. Banish all non-essential clocks from sight. Try to have a clock in only one room in the house, and position it so that it isn't readily visible. Use the clock on your mobile phone rather than a wristwatch – and keep it in your pocket or handbag.

◆ **Go back in time** Each week, pick one task or activity and decide to do it the old-fashioned way. Eat dinner by candlelight instead of turning on the lights. Walk to the shops to collect bread and milk rather than driving. Spend a quiet, pleasant hour picking out books at the local library, instead of surfing the Net for the information. All these activities help you to focus on the process as well as the outcome, and so heighten the pleasure of connecting to the moment.

21. EXPLORE YOUR WORLD

There is an old Chinese proverb that says, 'Every journey – great or small – starts with a single step.' Few things are as effective at helping you to find balance and feed your spirit as taking that first step out the door. A simple fifteen-minute walk in the fresh air raises your heart rate and improves circulation, and can greatly boost your mood, thanks to the release of feel-good hormones that put you in a calmer, more focused frame of mind.

Walking is not just a way of getting from point A to point B or even of turbo-charging your metabolism; it is a means of re-acquainting yourself with what's really important in your life and in your community. Try these ideas.

◆ **Wake up a bit earlier** Get up and enjoy the thrill of breathing fresh outdoor air before anyone else does. Notice how much more peaceful and centred you feel for the rest of the day.

◆ **Climb something** Find a water tower, a hill or the highest look-out point in your area. Take in the view from the top, look towards the horizon, and forget your worries.

◆ **Seek the new** Life is a journey, not a destination, as the saying goes. Rather than focus on where you're going, be mindful of what you see along the way. Next time you take a walk in a familiar area, set yourself the challenge of finding something new and unexpected along the way. You might notice a bright red front door or a shiny brass doorplate, an unusual shrub or tree. This exercise turns a simple walk around the block into a meditative exercise, making you focus on the moment and really notice your surroundings, rather than letting your mind race ahead to future commitments.

◆ **Wander off the beaten track** Try straying from your usual route. Be stimulated by new neighbourhoods and people, and appreciate the challenge of finding your way home.

◆ **Find the four elements** Balance your subtle inner energies and feel more in harmony with your surroundings by finding a place on your walk where you can experience all four elements: earth, air, water and fire. For example, you could walk on the grass (earth) near a fountain or creek (air and water) while enjoying the sensation of the sun (fire) on your face and body.

◆ **Walk with gratitude** As you walk, think of all the things you're grateful for in your life: happy, healthy children; a warm bed; friends who stand by you; a bird swooping overhead. Repeat the thought either in your head or out loud as a mantra, e.g. 'Thank you for the beautiful bird', or 'I'm so glad the boys have a sunny afternoon for tennis practice'. Sounds simplistic, but forcing your brain to focus on positive and meaningful connections in your life is one of the easiest ways to calm down and regain perspective. It's impossible to feel scattered and stressed when you are acknowledging all the things you're grateful for.

22. LEARN THE NAMES OF PLANTS

For centuries, the simplest way to dehumanise individuals was to take away their name. Sometimes this has been a shameful exercise, such as the ghastly tattooing of numbers on concentration camp inmates' arms. It can also be seen in the widespread custom of calling soldiers by their surname rather than their given name.

Putting a name to a face is essential to recognising and respecting that person as an individual. The same principle applies to the natural kingdom. By learning the names of birds, flowers and trees, you are paying them respect, honouring them as individual living things, and therefore able to establish a more meaningful connection with them.

Identifying some of the birds, flowers and trees that are native to your area is also a way to spark your interest in the natural world and to feel a stronger connection to your own territory. It changes the way you look at what surrounds you, and makes you more mindful and conscious of the things you see every day.

Being able to say, 'That's a beautiful rubra frangipani', for instance, and paying tribute to its unique make-up, creates a richer, more intimate experience than saying, 'That flower smells nice'. Giving something its particular name makes the world a fuller, more welcoming place, a place where you feel as though you belong.

23. MAKE POTPOURRI

Potpourri is a lovely traditional way to fill a room with the scent of flowers all year round. It's easy and fun to make your own – the ingredients are readily available from health-food stores and craft shops. Some Internet suppliers will even home-deliver.

As you scoop, measure, sift and stir, inhale the relaxing natural fragrance. Pour your finished blend into a beautiful china or glazed ceramic bowl and place it where it is sure to catch your eye – on the hallstand, perhaps, or on your bedside table. Whenever you pass by, trail your fingers in the mix: this releases a burst of fragrance, and reminds you of the pleasure you experienced when making it.

LEMON POTPOURRI

1 tablespoon dried lemon verbena
1 tablespoon dried lemon balm
1 tablespoon dried lemon thyme
3 dried bay leaves, crumbled
1 tablespoon dried lemon zest
2 tablespoons dried marigold petals or small yellow everlasting daisies
few drops neroli and/or orange essential oils

◆ Combine the dried leaves and zest in a large non-metallic bowl and mix well with your hands, enjoying the different textures as they flow through your fingers.

◆ Add the essential oils, a drop at a time, until your ideal level of fragrance is reached.

24. PUT DOWN ROOTS

'To understand where you are going,' says the Celtic proverb, 'you must understand where you have come from.'

What does 'home' mean to you? Perhaps you've just moved into a brand-new apartment, or maybe your family has lived in the same area or even in the same house for generations. Whether home is in a tiny town or in the middle of a city, the most reassuring thing about it is that you belong there, and that you have somewhere you can go where you are able to relax and just be yourself. It is the place where you belong.

To look at a street name or a farmhouse or a bridge and to have a sense of when it came to be there and why, and to know a little about the people who built or named it, brings stability and peace. Visit your local museum or council library one Saturday afternoon or during a lunch-hour. These places are a treasure trove of maps, deeds, site surveys and charts. The caretakers are often older volunteers, and they love nothing more than to tell you how things were in their day.

It's fascinating to learn that the one-way street you drive down each morning on the way to work used to be a tannery ... or that the netball court at the local school was the site of a bomb shelter during World War II ... or that Rosedale Avenue was so named because there was a market garden there, famous for its roses ... or that the 'Sarah' of Sarah's Lookout was a young woman whose fiancé was killed in an accident, and who spent her days thereafter sadly walking along the foreshore at that spot ... or that the ornate wrought-iron gates at the entrance to the local park were salvaged from the first farmhouse built in your area 150 years ago, long since demolished.

Poring over dusty glass cabinets containing photographs of long-dead soldiers and schoolchildren, newspaper clippings and letters in spidery handwriting is a powerful exercise in gaining perspective. You see your surroundings in a fresh light and feel a connection to the history of everyday human experience – these people were just like you.

25. GIVE SOMETHING BACK

'Do not care overly much for wealth, power or fame,' wrote Rudyard Kipling. 'One day you will meet someone who cares for none of these things and you will realise how poor you have become.'

Peace of mind is definitely not about what – or how much – you get in life, it's about what you give back. Voluntary work and charitable activities enhance happiness, self-esteem, a sense of control, physical health and depression relief, all of which contribute to significantly redressing the balance of personal wellbeing and life satisfaction in your favour.

We all have so much to offer – money, love, ideas, elbow grease and expertise. However, even if your income is less than you'd like it to be, giving of your time will make you feel truly rich and generous. Use the gift of giving to make a difference to someone else's life, and to deepen your own sense of self-worth. Psychologists call this side-effect of helping others 'elevation' – the uplifting feeling you get when you do a really kind act, as though your heart is opening. Doing something for others also helps to minimise the effects of the ongoing, free-floating anxiety in our post-9/11 world. For example, researchers have found that volunteers who gave money and donated blood after the Bali bombings were better able to overcome their shock and anger. Consider the following ideas.

◆ **Volunteer at a soup kitchen or homeless shelter** Even just an hour or two every six weeks can make a difference to people who truly need support.

◆ **Help out at a wildlife rescue centre** Often an injured animal's life depends on having someone at the end of a hotline who can collect them, and take them to a veterinary service outside of regular hours.

◆ **Support your local school or sheltered workshop** These places rely heavily on volunteers to paint rooms, fix gardens, donate old toys, clothing or recyclable materials, and much more.

26. CREATE RIPPLES

Mother Teresa said, 'Be faithful to the small things: punctuality, words of kindness, a thought for others, your way of looking, of speaking and of acting.' It is these small things in life that present us with opportunities to make a strong and authentic connection with the world around us, to break through boundaries and to experience closer contact with other humans, to feel reassured and in touch.

Decide to be a force for the positive in your world, and to make active, joyous connections with others. Positive relationships aren't gifts – they're the result of habits. Instead of reflexively seeing the worst, focus on the beauty and goodness in people and events. This doesn't mean false flattery or political correctness, nor does it mean ignoring danger signals. What it does mean is finding the good in relationships and trying to improve difficult ones.

Imagine you have tossed a pebble into a still pond, and you are watching the ripples spread out, further and further. The same principle applies to you – your smallest action or word can have profoundly far-reaching effects. Seek opportunities to pay compliments, offer praise or give a helping hand every single day. Showing kindness in any circumstance is the greatest compliment you can offer another person. Here are some ideas for creating positive life-ripples that recharge your spirit and create new connections between you and your world.

♦ **Give a reason** Tell the people whom you love why you love them. Say 'I care about you because you ...' or 'You matter to me because ...' Say it out loud, don't expect them to guess.

♦ **Praise other people's abilities** Say to the postman or the garage mechanic, 'You're doing a great job' – magic words that can make a person's day. Move on to your co-workers or friends.

♦ **Compliment a stranger** Tell someone that you just love their haircut, handbag or shoes. Walking past a mum with a baby in a stroller? Say, 'Oh, isn't she beautiful!' and smile.

- **Reach out and touch** Gently pat a colleague's hand when you thank them for giving you information. Never pass up an opportunity to give someone a congratulatory slap on the shoulder or an affectionate squeeze.

- **Show good manners** Nearly 200 years ago, Ralph Waldo Emerson wrote, 'There is always time for courtesy.' It doesn't matter if you're a man or a woman; opening doors, pulling out chairs, offering another person the next place in the queue are all easy ways to make someone else's day, and improve yours.

- **Say 'thank you'** Acknowledge everyone, whether they are young or old, fast or slow, family members or complete strangers. The simplest expression of gratitude is a gift to the giver as well as the recipient.

- **Play the game 'New or Good'** At the end of each day, ask your partner or child to tell you about one new or good experience they've had. Then offer your own response. Maybe you noticed blooming pink roses or a flock of bright green parrots or your cranky neighbour smiled.

- **Sparkle** 'Be the change you wish to see in the world,' said Mahatma Gandhi. For one week, try to make his advice come alive by sprinkling some positive 'fairy dust' on everything that you do. Be enthusiastic and bright at the office. Recognise people, remember their names and use them often – no one likes to be ignored. Smile and speak pleasantly to others. Tell jokes. Watch how others respond to you.

27. KEEP IT REAL

Faced with constant pressure to buy more clothes, more CDs and more stuff in general, it's easy to lose sight of the pleasure to be found in giving a real present to someone, and then watching their face light up because they just love it.

In fact, up until Victorian times, expensive store-bought presents were only for the privileged few; instead, the main emphasis was on distributing food and money to the poor. If you want to make a more meaningful connection with a gift, think of ideas that reflect your relationship with that person.

◆ **Give of yourself** Pass on your own possessions to people you love, e.g. a favourite book, a treasured ring, a framed sketch or painting that reflects an aspect of your relationship or shared history.

◆ **Do things together** Make a date for a day together – attending a workshop, pottering around an antiquarian bookstore, taking a bushwalk.

◆ **Share real entertainment** Instead of catching a movie together, treat yourself to a live show. It doesn't have to be expensive – there are plenty of free community discussion panels, stand-up comedy reviews and local band recitals on offer. Skipping electronic entertainment gives you a chance to engage with the players in a spontaneous, energetic way that just doesn't happen with an edited, pre-taped show or a movie where the gags and storylines that have been researched and analysed to the nth degree.

◆ **Create a memorable experience** Give them a special activity that they wouldn't otherwise get around to doing themselves – a wine-tasting, a flight in a hot-air balloon, an introductory class (belly-dancing, snorkelling, self-defence, Thai cookery or tai chi), a ride through the city streets in a horse-drawn carriage or a trip to the dog-races.

◆ **A photograph album** Collate photos of times shared with that person.

◆ **A box of dress-up clothes** Old nighties, wild shoes, silly ties, outrageous costume jewellery, cute hats – all can provide hours of fun and creative play for a child.

28. GO FOR A WALK WITH A CHILD

'Know you what it is to be a child?' asked the poet Percy Bysshe Shelley. 'It is to believe in the power of belief itself; it is to turn pumpkins into coaches, and mice into horses, and nothing into everything.' Most grown-ups who are busy earning a living, commuting and doing household chores have lost – or at the very least mislaid – the fascination and curiosity about their natural surroundings that they had as children.

To rekindle that sense of wonder, go for a walk in the park or along a beach with a small child. The first thing you will notice is that your pace will become slower: children can dawdle along for hours, looking at everything and nothing. They stop to squat down and poke a stick at a caterpillar or to pick up a feather, a leaf, a shell fragment or a rock with an interesting shape.

Even if you both only walk to the end of your street and back, the child will see something wonderful – 'Look at that cat in the window!' – or find a new mystery in a winged seedpod or a dragonfly.

When you look at the world through a child's eyes, there are magical treasures everywhere. Trace the pattern of bark on a tree. Listen to a gutter full of leaves and gurgling brown water after a downpour. Lie flat on your back on the grass and watch the clouds overhead: see if you can make out shapes of a lion, a dragon, a letterbox. Turn a stone over with the toe of your shoe and watch the earwigs scuttle away. Hunker down and peer closer: put a crumb on the ground and wait and watch until an ant picks up that boulder of a crumb and hauls it away.

If you care about birds, beetles and flowers, you will always be able to tap into your childlike sense of wonder, and you will never have a boring or stressful day again, because even the tiniest experience can seem like a miracle.

29. COLLECT TREASURE

What does the word 'beauty' mean to you? We are conditioned to define beauty as something that is perfect, lovely, stylish, but also often larger than life, impressive and glamorous. To appreciate the natural wonder in the world around you, it is necessary to look beyond this definition of beauty, and to notice the small and exquisite ordinary things that touch your heart.

A walk along a bush path or a creek bed can yield the most extraordinary collection of beautiful things – a piece of cuttlefish, a prickly seedcase, a piece of amber glass polished smooth by many years of being tossed and tumbled in the sea and sand, a bird's feather, tipped with electric blue.

Collecting these talismans and keeping them in a special treasure box is a way of focusing your senses so that you pause to look around you at the natural world, to listen and feel. It's also a link to childhood, and of days spent beachcombing and cubby-making, and when you would bring home a shell or rock to keep and look at more closely in the privacy of your room.

Perhaps you already have a suitable box. If you don't, buy one from a craft shop and decorate it in a way that's meaningful to you.

TREASURE BOX

> a selection of small shells, pebbles or flattish stones
> craft glue
> small lidded wooden box
> clear varnish

◆ Glue the shells, pebbles or stones all over the box and lid in a decorative pattern, leaving the area where the lid slides down onto the box free.

◆ Set the box aside until the glue dries, then paint it with clear varnish.

30. MAKE LEAF RUBBINGS

Leaves mark the natural rhythm of the seasons – soft new green leaves in spring; bold, rich gold and red in autumn; crackling underfoot in winter. Collecting leaves can be a mini-meditation on change and on celebrating differences, because they come in so many shapes and sizes. Pick a handful of different leaves and look at them very closely – at the textures and patterns, the colours and flaws – and at how incredibly beautiful they are.

You can have some very simple, satisfying, creative fun by making leaf rubbings.

LEAF RUBBINGS

> a few large pieces of paper
> selection of different leaves (those with contrasting and distinctive outlines and rib patterns will work best)
> wax crayons or charcoal

◆ Arrange the leaves on one piece of paper, then place another sheet over the top. Secure the sides with a few pieces of sticky tape, if you like.

◆ Run a wax crayon or stick of charcoal lightly over the top of the paper from side to side, covering the whole piece of paper, so that the leaves' shapes come through as rubbings.

31. CLEAR AWAY STALE ENERGY

Many native cultures have in common the view that everything in the world is filled with spiritual energy drawn from a universal power. It follows that everything is connected on an energetic level – air, earth, water, rocks, trees, animals, humans – in the great cycle of life.

So we are faced with a choice: we can either distance ourselves from this natural state and try to control or dominate it, or we can embrace it, and try to embody the spirit or essence in ourselves. One Native American tradition for restoring energetic balance is smudging – or burning – of special herbs, usually sage.

Buy a smudge stick from your health-food store. Light it as you would an incense stick and walk through your home, allowing the sweet-smelling smoke to fill the rooms. As you do so, say 'With this smoke, I will clear away negative energy.' Welcome the spirit and scent of nature into your home, and be grateful for the spirit forces all around you.

If a smudge stick doesn't appeal, note that decorating with freshly cut greenery does more than just add a touch of colour to your home. In pagan times, villagers cut branches of evergreen trees, such as pine and juniper, and brought them indoors during the cold months because they believed they were home to powerful spirits.

The scent, shape and texture of many everyday trees and shrubs such as eucalyptus, ferns, ivy and cypress work wonders on your mind and body. The scent of eucalyptus, for instance, is a mood lifter and a relaxant, while cypress is a nerve tonic and can help you feel more tranquil.

No flowers in your garden to pick? Just snip a few lengths of graceful greenery, then sit back and admire their calming presence.

32. GROW HYACINTHS

There is an Taoist proverb which says that if you lose all your worldly goods except for two coins, you should use one to buy bread to feed your body, and the other to buy hyacinths to feed your soul. Hyacinths have the most exquisitely sweet, cool and delicate perfume. Keep a pot on your desk or dining table, and you will feel your spirits lift every time you look at them.

Other bulbs suitable for growing indoors are crocus, freesia, galanthus, narcissus, dwarf iris and tulips. All are easy to grow and may be persuaded to flower in midwinter, their bright colours reminding you that spring will return.

The best way to obtain gorgeous, long-lasting flowers from potted bulbs is to follow the old-timers' trick and start them off in the dark. Follow the directions below and then place the pot inside a dark cupboard, or cover it with a few sheets of newspaper, or upend another pot of a similar size and put it on top.

GROWING BULBS

> compost or bulb fibre
> a shallow bowl
> bulbs
> potting mix and compost

◆ Put a layer of compost or special bulb fibre in the bottom of a bowl.

◆ Set the bulbs in the bowl as close together as you can. It does not matter if they touch each other.

◆ Carefully fill up the spaces between the bulbs with potting mix and compost, pressing down firmly between them until the container is almost full. Moisten the compost slightly, but do not soak. The neck of big bulbs like hyacinths or daffodils can be left sticking out the top; smaller ones should be covered.

◆ Put the bowls in a cool, dark room for six weeks. Keep moist but not soggy at all times.

◆ When the leaf shoots reach about 10 cm, bring the bowl into a room that gets natural light or place on a windowsill.

33. BE VERY QUIET

Being constantly on the move, hurrying and rushing towards goals, does not allow you time for thinking and just being, which are the states that give your brain the best chance of working out rational and sensible responses to stressful situations or people. The Dalai Lama describes this behaviour as 'being very busy practising superficialities'.

Many of the repetitive activities that take up your day, such as constantly checking email, are not essential. They can, paradoxically, be just as stressful as doing too little. Being constantly busy is a type of addiction, leaving you dissatisfied, restless and numb. It also increases your heart rate and your body's production of cortisol (the stress hormone), and interferes with your ability to concentrate. Even if you're not rushing around, extraneous noise can overstimulate your nerves, slowing the amount of information coming into your brain.

According to the proverb, 'Silence is golden'. So every day, pencil in at least one ten-minute break for complete silence. Seek out a corner away from others where you can be perfectly still and quiet. Switch off the fax and your mobile phone. If you're at home, turn off the washing machine and dryer. Shut down your computer, walk away and sit down in a quiet room. Close your eyes and listen for everyday 'real' noises instead – the birds outside, the chatter of children walking home from school, even an ice-cream van. Then, when you feel more at peace, turn everything back on and get back to work. Silence is the ultimate time-out, and even a few minutes' worth can be astonishingly restorative, helping you to calm down and think clearly. As you sit quietly, check into the stillness at your centre. See what happens in the silence.

34. OR, MAKE A LOT OF NOISE

What do loud rock 'n' roll music and Native American tribal rituals, gospel services and full-moon raves in Bali all have in common? Lots of noise and lots of movement, usually to the powerful rhythm of drums.

In the West, we have traditionally viewed depressed mood states such as anger, rage and frustration, as things that have to be subdued or controlled. Consider the usual prescription of painkillers or sedatives, and the advice to 'calm down' or even to lie still and rest in bed. This dulling of the senses can actually worsen some people's feelings of isolation and disconnection. Eastern and native cultures, on the other hand, especially the African, Hawaiian and Caribbean traditions, prescribe vigorous movement to a pounding rhythm. Native shamen pound drums and lead tribe members in wild, stomping, free-form dances to celebrate the seasons, drive away evil spirits and pacify the gods.

Drumming has a transcendent power. Possibly the most ancient of all musical sounds, it is a link to our primal selves, our fundamental nature. The physical act of thumping a drum with your hands or a pair of sticks improves your mood by releasing tension. And, if you can drum to the point that you are totally absorbed by the noise and the rhythm and oblivious to everything else that's happening around you, then you're in the same still and clear state of mind that you can achieve with meditation.

Many health clubs offer tribal dance classes, accompanied by traditional drummers. Or, buy your own drum from a music or New Age store.

35. LISTEN TO THE WIND

Many centuries ago the Greeks made beautifully carved wind chimes from cedarwood and pipes of beaten brass. They placed them in the windows and doorways of their homes and temples, where the chimes caught the breeze and played evocative, magical music.

To soothe your senses, relax your mind and connect with the natural world, not much beats sitting under a leafy tree and watching the first stars of evening appear, while listening to the sound of a warm breeze flirting with a wind chime.

Buy a wind chime and hang it high up in a tree, or near a door or hallway where it will catch the breeze. When you hear it play, think about the nature of the wind: it can be strong enough to rattle windows or even blow roofs off houses, yet soft enough to barely tickle your face and lift your hair off your neck. You, too, are strong and determined – and yet you have the capacity to be playful, gentle and surprising. Listen to your wind chime's beautiful, ever-changing melody, and imagine yourself moving and adapting, dipping and swaying in life's dance.

36. GO OUTSIDE AND PLAY

Up, up, up on a swing, up in the air so blue … Every child has thought that, if they can just manage one more big push while on a swing, they will be able to reach the sky. Swings are perennial favourites with children, but there's no rule that says stressed, jaded, out-of-touch adults can't hop aboard and be liberated from the relentless round of work cares.

A swing is one of the simplest and most relaxing pleasures life has to offer. Parks and playgrounds often provide swings that you can visit at lunch-time, or you can easily rig up your own in your backyard if you have a sturdy tree. No tree? You can purchase a swing with a metal or wooden frame in kit form, which you can assemble and bolt together yourself.

No garden? Buy a swing chair for your porch, terrace or balcony, one of the old-fashioned ones with a canopy. Curl up on the seat, and rock gently to and fro. Lazing on a swing brings quick relief from the cares of the world and is the epitome of lazy, languid Sunday afternoons when you should have nothing to do except read a little and eat and doze a lot.

Better yet – if you have the courage – slide down a hill, and get grass stains all over the back of your pants.

Find a sturdy cardboard box – preferably one that's at least 6 mm thick. Cut out the base of the box; this will give you a sled-like piece large enough to sit on with your knees bent, your hands holding on to the front edge. Climb up a nice green hillside and then slide down.

Or just lie on the grass, horizontal to the fall of the hill, and flip yourself over – and over – and over – as you roll and bump your way down. Smell the earth, get bits of grass in your hair, and whoop till you're breathless. Your heart's racing – what a blast!

37. GO CAMPING

Imagine you have just arrived at a camping site for the weekend. What's the first thing that you notice when you get out and look around? The incredible QUIET. No phones, no television, no constant hum of electrical appliances.

Getting away from so-called civilisation is a marvellous way to relax and to restore your sense of balance. Escaping the cars, buildings, cement, people and all their attendant noise and demands guarantees a drop in blood pressure and a new perspective on what's important in your life. Being outside in nature encourages you to look around with fresh eyes, to switch off your everyday mind.

Find peace camping by a mountain creek, in the desert or near the ocean. Wear soft old T-shirts and baggy pants; leave the hairdryer, make-up and high-heeled shoes behind. Enjoy peaceful days without hearing a single mechanical sound, just the call of birds and the rhythm of your own footsteps. Get in touch with the silence within yourself and know that everything in life has a purpose. Food tastes better, the sun feels warmer, and you'll sleep better than you ever do at home.

38. HAVE A VISION

Having a vision statement can help you cut through meaningless activity, and focus only on those things that will energise you and feed your spirit.

Draw three columns on a piece of paper. Head each with the following: 'I am', 'I want' and 'I can'. Now, write down the answers, using the active, present tense. For example, 'I am a hard-working, loyal person. I want peace of mind and the calm satisfaction that comes from knowing that I have done my best. I can make a difference in my life and in other people's lives.'

Now, hold yourself to this one, articulated decision. Tape it to your fridge door or use it as your screensaver. This one-decision–one-vision technique is different from serial goal-setting. It's your quest for yourself and it helps you realise you can be more than you are. A vision statement makes you feel more alive, prompting you to rise to the occasion when you least expect it. When a step has to be taken, take it: there is no one totally right time for anything.

39. BLESS YOURSELF

In a world of rap lyrics, phonetic spelling and general 'dumbing down', we are not as familiar as we once were with the profound and inspiring effects of language. It is ironic that, on the one hand, we have in common a deep hunger for meaningful connection, a need for the calm and comfort that words can provide, but on the other, we are often frustrated by an inability to communicate.

This is particularly true for those of us who are uncomfortable or unfamiliar with the formal rituals offered by organised religions, yet who nonetheless crave the feeling of community and inspiration found in spiritual practice. Learning a simple blessing can go a long way towards satisfying this hunger and restoring the sense of 'God being in His heaven, all's right with the world' that Elizabeth Barrett Browning wrote of.

Blessings can be found in a variety of writing, spiritual and secular. One of the most deceptively powerful, simple phrases I have ever read is this ancient Celtic prayer: 'All will be well, and all will be well, and all will be well.' To me, this is a blessing, a grace, a mantra and a comfort, all rolled into one.

Find a line or a phrase that is meaningful to you. Learn it off by heart and use it often during the day as a soothing benediction before eating or leaving the house, perhaps, or as you wake and when you lie down to sleep. Use it often. Here are some ideas to get you started.

Don't think about the future; just be here now. Don't think about the past; just be here now. (Ram Dass)

To every thing there is a season, and a time to every purpose under heaven. (Ecclesiastes 3:1–4)

Shanti, shanti, shanti. (*Peace, peace, peace* – traditional Vedic prayer.

40. MAKE FRIENDS OF ALL AGES

John Lennon wrote that in the end the love you take is equal to the love you make. It is important for your long-term mental wellbeing and physical health to have a wide circle of friends. Researchers have found that people with few or unsatisfactory personal relationships have four times the risk of early death as those with an active social life and satisfying friendships, even when other factors such as diet and exercise were considered.

Most often, your friends will be around the same age as you and probably share similar experiences, such as work choices or children. However, recognise that this will not always be the case: a friend does not have to be someone like you, he or she just has to be someone who likes you. It can be a boy or a girl, a teacher or a neighbour. Stop hurrying and rushing so fast and look around to notice the person who smiles at you in a certain way, or the child who prefers to sit next to you and let you be quiet.

For example, I treasured my friendship with my mother's friend Kath, who was full of wry wisdom and always keen on discussing issues and exploring new ideas even though she was forty years older than me. I also love being friends with Miki, whose remarkably sensible, clear-eyed observations belie the fact that she's only nine years old.

Having friends of all ages helps you to grow by providing different perspectives on life. If people have drifted away, join a professional association, book group or craft class to find people with whom you have something in common.

41. PUT IT IN WRITING

With the ease and accessibility of email and telephones, 'snail mail' has almost become a lost art. However, to sit and write even the briefest note or card by hand is a chance to make a much deeper and more intimate connection with another person. It's a chance to express how you feel and to bring people together, both of which are critical to developing stress hardiness and a more balanced life.

Use these simple rituals to reach out to others in a tangible way, and to give and receive love.

◆ **Write notes** Use your best pen and stationery.

◆ **Remember birthdays** Write a letter or draw up a long scroll listing favourite memories of a friend and what they mean to you. Send it to them for their birthday.

◆ **Add a little extra** If you give someone a book, write a brief dedication on the front flap. Same goes for a poster or a painting.

42. GO GOOGLE

For many years, mine was only a very small family consisting of my mother and my two sons. So it was a delightful bonus when I married Doug to find that he was part of a fine, big family of interesting, affectionate and energetic people. The only hitch was, they didn't live in the same city as we did. Solution? Email.

Email messages are simple, inexpensive and lots of fun. It takes only minutes to prepare quick updates about what's been happening – it can be in point form, if you like – and, if you've got a digital camera, you can attach a couple of recent happy snaps. You could even set up your own website and post photos, jokes and news.

The Internet is also a way of tracking down old friends and family members. Perhaps there was a falling out or one of you just moved away. Whatever the reason why you lost touch in the first place, catching up can be a delightful surprise.

The only way to have friends is to be one. Invest in the quality of your relationships and show others that you care by creating a cyberworld where you can stay in touch. Reconnecting helps heal old wounds, expands your vision and gives you a fresh perspective on your life. Sharing stories of life's experiences with an old friend is a measuring stick, and helps you to acknowledge what you've achieved, and how far you've come since you last saw each other. You may find that, quite suddenly, you are able to let go of a grudge you've had for twenty years. And even if the reunion isn't one you want to pursue, it may be a reality check – perhaps the lesson is to let that person go and free up those thoughts and emotions so you can invest them in other relationships.

A friend is a present you give yourself. So go Google an old friend, and see where the experience leads you.

43. SAY 'I LOVE YOU' EVERY DAY

My friend Louella was diagnosed with terminal cancer at fifty-two. 'Nasty. Inoperable. You've got twelve weeks. Put your affairs in order,' said the oncologist, with an abominable lack of compassion. She defied him then, standing up in his office, with her green eyes blazing. And she continued to defy him and his prognosis for a further four years.

Lou said that the only thing that kept her going was her love for her children. Over the next four years she said over and over, 'I can't die, I can't leave the kids, I've got to look after my kids.' She loved those children with the most enormous, awe-inspiring love, the kind that doesn't die, even after the person has gone. And they loved her back.

When I was twenty, I believed in 'true love' – a vision made up of a man in a dinner suit who would write sonnets about me in romantic settings, and feed me handmade truffles and champagne. In short, all the symbols of feelings as defined by other people (usually selling those chocolates and champagne).

Now I am forty, and Lou has taught me that the greatest affection is given – and received – without expectations. It's in the cross-eyed clay elephant Ed made for me; it's in the desk calendar from Randall, with the picture pasted on upside-down; it's in a look, a gesture, a touch, a 'Well done, I'm so proud of you' from Mum. These quieter rituals are the things that give us the strength, comfort and security that we need to go back into the world, day after day.

I miss Lou, but I am grateful for her gift to me: she showed me that the only way to be loved is to love with abandon. Without love, life is a dry and heartless exercise. With it, your soul is nourished and your spirit soars. Every day, tell the people who matter to you that you love and appreciate them. And love your children unconditionally, no matter how messy their rooms are, how many exams they fail, how rude their friends are or how many lies they tell. Tell them you love them every day.

44. LOOK UP AT THE NIGHT SKY

'Teach me your mood, patient stars! Who climb each night the ancient sky, leaving no shade, no scars, no trace of age, no fear to die,' wrote Ralph Waldo Emerson. Like Emerson, generations of humans have stood silently beneath the stars on a clear night and looked up, wondering about the ancient, fathomless universe and their place in it. It is humbling to contemplate the endless distances and infinite potential of space, and to realise what a very tiny part you have in it.

Gazing at the night sky makes you feel more connected to the natural world. It also gives you a sense of the passage of time. The Native American Cree Indians have an expression, 'I am the reason why my ancestors existed.'

Go outside before bedtime and look up at the stars. Focus on one and just breathe quietly. Imagine your parents, your grandparents and generations of ancestors all flowing back and away, into time and space. These people are all around you, a part of the earth and sky, and a part of your body's cells and unique spirit. Give thanks for your life and realise how insignificant your own problems really are.

Then make a wish. Star light, star bright, first star I see tonight … Close your eyes, take ten deep breaths and imagine yourself letting go. Trust in the Universe. Trust in yourself.

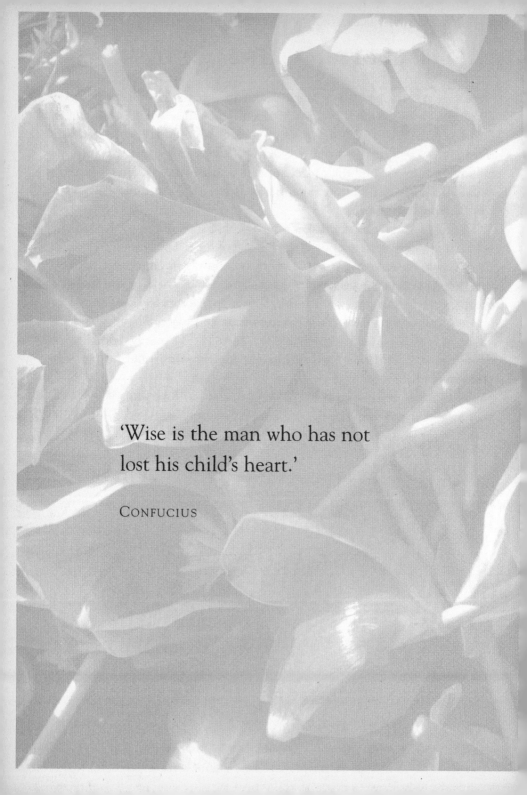

'Wise is the man who has not
lost his child's heart.'

CONFUCIUS

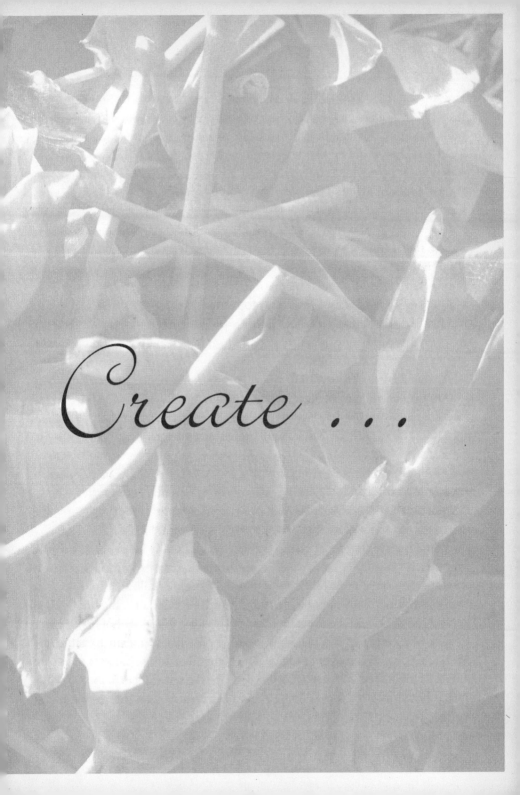

Create . . .

Doing something creative and enjoyable is a shortcut to feeling calm, and leaves you uplifted, happy and 'juiced'. It can be as simple as lying on the grass watching the clouds drift overhead, or taking a different route to work. Or it could be a hobby like learning the drums, growing orchids or making mosaics, or a long-held dream to build a house, take up horse-riding or see the pyramids of Egypt. Think back to activities you've enjoyed in the past – sports, crafts, drama – and look for clues.

Creativity is also about what you choose not to do. You may decide to reduce television viewing – or at least only watch programs that inspire you – and in its place choose instead to read, do a jigsaw or learn a language. Take a long, hard look at popular recreational activities that subtract, rather than add, meaning, and that do nothing to restore balance to your life. Drifting around the shopping complex, playing video games and trawling gossip magazines for the latest news on Paris Hilton may seem restful and pleasant, but in fact are just numbing you.

Truly creative activities will nourish, inspire and energise you, and help you to find balance in two ways. First, they're fun. Remember 'All work and no play makes Jack a dull boy'? No play makes us worse than dull – it makes us dead. Doing without breaks and simple pleasures reduces your ability to fight disease and takes a toll on energy levels.

Secondly, doing something creative helps you to shift your perspective and use your mind. Creative stimulation actually grows new brain connections and strengthens old ones, thus boosting your memory and strengthening your mental capacity to cope with future stress.

Sometimes a change in creative direction can really be as good as a rest, whether it's a small change such as throwing a party or writing a poem, a medium one such as enrolling for a course of study or taking a fresh look at the way you normally approach an aspect of your work, or a big one such as repainting the house, moving, or going on holiday. Boredom is a major cause of lack of creative energy, whereas focusing on what you want to achieve – setting goals, checking your progress and generally taking charge of your own life – are great creative energisers. A good tip is to remember that worthwhile goals should involve you in doing something creative and interesting rather than waiting for something to happen to you: being active gives you momentum. The reason that many people find it difficult to give up an energy-draining habit, such as constantly worrying and focusing on their problems, is because all their energies are directed towards *not* doing something.

Incorporate more play in your day and you'll be happier, more productive, and have higher self-esteem. A creative activity doesn't have to be big or challenging, nor do you have to do it perfectly. The trick is to lose yourself in the process, to be completely absorbed in a task, even if it's for just a short time. Nor do the activities have to be planned; keep things spontaneous, fun and simple.

45. BUILD A BIRDBATH

When the boys were small, the three of us planned to spend a Saturday afternoon building a birdbath and planting flowers around it. Well, honesty bids me tell you that the boys drifted off halfway through, leaving me to finish the job. Hot and very cross, I went inside to clean myself up. 'Mummy, Mummy!' Randall shouted. Grimly, I put down the disinfectant and went into the garden. 'Isn't it great? Aren't they wonderful?' he exclaimed, his cornflower-blue eyes sparkling with excitement as two scarlet rosellas perched on the new birdbath.

Birds need water every day to survive. Besides drinking, birds also need water to wash themselves. To attract birds into your garden, balcony or courtyard, ensure there is a birdbath.

Simplest of all is a rock with a natural dent in it, or a ceramic or terracotta saucer placed on a stump or ledge out of reach of predators. You will find that once birds have been attracted by the water, they will want to stay and find something to eat. Set up a birdfeeder near the birdbath, and spend a few moments every day just enjoying the sight of the birds darting around and squabbling over titbits; you will automatically smile and feel calmer just watching them.

Another idea is to take a bag of breadcrumbs or unsalted nuts to a park. Imagine every crumb or nut is a problem. As you throw each one, name it and say, 'That gets rid of you!' Watch your worries get eaten up and disappear.

46. PRESS FLOWERS

Like many so-called 'children's games', pressing flowers and using them to make cards, stationery, bookmarks or even small pictures is a supremely relaxing hobby for adults, too.

The actions of collecting and arranging the flowers are simple and repetitive, which helps you to become absorbed in what you are doing. The process takes time, and so it teaches you patience, and gives you a sense of being in touch with natural, unforced rhythms. And making a batch of cards and filing them away for future use also gives you a great sense of satisfaction and accomplishment – friends and family will value that personal touch.

The easiest way to start is to place individual flowers between sheets of clean blotting paper and then put them between the pages of a heavy book, such as the telephone directory. Place more weights such as bricks or books on top.

You can buy small flower presses from craft shops and garden centres. Leave the flowers for 4–6 weeks, then check to see if they are ready to use.

PRESSED FLOWER CARDS

◆ Fold sheets of paper or light card in half.

◆ On a separate piece of paper, set out the pressed flowers in a design – perhaps as a circle, a heart or initials.

◆ When you are satisfied with the design, start to pick up the individual pieces, and apply a little glue to the backs of the flowers and petals with the point of a toothpick.

◆ Fix the flowers into place on the front of the card. When they are correctly positioned, press down on them with a clean piece of paper to set them in place. Leave the glue to set properly before putting the cards in envelopes.

47. BAKE BROWNIES

It's not possible to remain in a sour mood if you're making a sweet treat. Cooking can be a very settling and relaxing thing to do, especially if you're making this luscious brownie. There is no serious purpose to it, nutritional or otherwise; you're creating something just for the sheer joy of it. And there is a secret, sinful delight in enjoying the sensuous foreplay to actually eating a brownie – filling your kitchen with that delectable, come-hither chocolate scent, leisurely licking the spoon and running your finger around the bowl to get the last traces of the mixture, then finally biting into the warm, chewy crust.

BROWNIES

⅓ cup plain (all-purpose) flour
½ cup cocoa powder
2 cups caster sugar
1 cup chopped pecans
250 g (8 oz) good-quality dark cooking chocolate
250 g (8 oz) butter
2 teaspoons vanilla essence
2–3 eggs, lightly beaten

♦ Preheat the oven to 180°C (350°F). Lightly grease a 20 x 30 cm (8 x 12 in) cake tin. Line the base and sides with baking paper.

♦ Sift the flour and cocoa into a bowl and add the sugar and nuts. Mix together and make a well in the centre. Grate the chocolate, or chop finely in a food processor, and add to the dry ingredients.

♦ Melt the butter in a small pan over a low heat, and add to the dry ingredients with the vanilla and eggs. Mix well.

♦ Pour into the tin, smooth the surface and bake for 50 minutes. Do not overcook. The top will crack and the mixture should still be a bit soft on the inside.

♦ Cool on a wire rack and refrigerate for at least 2 hours before cutting and serving. Brownies freeze well.

48. START A COLLECTION

A collection is so intensely personal. I have known people with collections of teapots, Toby jugs, ruby glass, antique corkscrews, china owls, salt-and-pepper shakers, toy penguins, thimbles, Victorian toy trains, Christmas tree ornaments, dolls, watches, pens, champagne glasses, odd keys and chocolate wrappers. The collections all have one thing in common: they tell a story. As the collector picks up an item or points it out to describe it to you, she will say something like, 'Now, I found this when I was …'

A collection may be worth a lot of money, but its true value is measured by the creative pleasure you gain from it, and the satisfaction you get from the absorbing activity of collecting itself, the way it acts as a record of your emotions and experiences over a long period of time – perhaps your whole life. Pretty soon your collection will be the inspiration for the gifts you get for birthdays and Christmas, until you're known simply as 'the frog lady' or 'the guy with all the 78 records' or 'the woman with all the 1920s powder compacts' (that's me).

Collecting gives you a sense of continuity in your life that is deeply soothing and reassuring. There are no pressures. You don't have to add to your collection every day, nor do you need to seek out new additions by a deadline. Half the pleasure of adding something new to a collection comes from finding the item in a place you never would have expected. An ordinary day suddenly becomes 'the day that you were driving back from dropping the kids at band camp, when you suddenly noticed …'

A collection might even prompt you to take new paths you would never have otherwise taken. After years of collecting first editions of books just for the pleasure of it, my grandfather moved into a business selling antiquarian books and maps – a byway he had not previously considered.

49. GROW STRAWBERRIES

'Shall I not have intelligence with the earth? Am I not partly leaves and vegetable mould myself?' asked author Henry David Thoreau over 150 years ago.

Thoreau wrote widely and poignantly on the subject of the earth's seasons and rhythms, and of the importance of living in harmony with Nature's laws. Any gardener will know what he meant – every garden is a reminder that everything flows and changes, that nothing stays the same, and that living things lean towards the light in order to grow. No wonder gardeners are among the sanest, kindest and most well-balanced people you will ever meet.

Gardening also teaches you that, no matter how upset or stressed you are, the smell of freshly turned earth can put things in perspective once more. Even the smallest garden-in-a-jar – like this strawberry pot – serves as a three-step mini meditation. First, in the planting and preparation; secondly, in watching the plants grow; and thirdly, in your looking after it. As with every relationship, the more caring, mindful and noticing you are, the greater the return to you.

STRAWBERRY POT

Strawberries are beautiful and delicious; they are also extremely decorative and easy to grow in special terracotta or earthenware strawberry planter pots. The pots are available in garden accessory shops and nurseries, along with punnets of ready-to-plant strawberry runners.

◆ Line the base with small stones or gravel to facilitate drainage. Fill the container with a good quality potting mix, forking through some compost as you go.

◆ Insert a strawberry plant in each opening in the pot, and fill the top of the container as well. Allow the runners to hang down and root in the openings, instead of being supported, so they appear to climb.

◆ Take a minute to water your planter pot daily – the little pockets do dry out rapidly. Pinch off a berry or three and treat yourself.

50. BLOW BUBBLES

We sat out on the back steps one Sunday afternoon, the boys and I, and blew beautiful iridescent wobbly soap bubbles. Randall whooped with delight, his turquoise-blue eyes sparkling, jumping and pointing and squealing, 'More, Mummy – more!'

Edward, older, serious-eyed, solemnly practised his bubble-blowing over and over till he made a simply enormous one, which floated up and up, almost over the top of the crepe myrtle tree.

Where has all the time gone? It's true what people say when you have babies – enjoy them, because they're only little for such a short time. Bubble-blowing on the back steps is one of many small treasured memories that I have of my sons – and I call it to mind every so often when I'm not sure I'm going to survive their adolescence.

Bubble-blowing is also a soothing, playful, whimsical thing to do whenever you feel like it, irrespective of how old you are. There is no point to it – which is the whole point! Keep an inexpensive bubble pipe in your kitchen drawer; dip it in a dish of soapy water and blow gently. Imagine all your cares floating away.

51. BUILD A TREE HOUSE

'I shall live with Tink,' declared Peter, 'in a little house we built for Wendy'. By building a tree house, you will be sharing Peter Pan's time-honoured secret escape. Tree houses have been used by generations of children, as well as by many famous people. Tarzan of the Apes, the Swiss Family Robinson and Winnie the Pooh all lived in tree houses, but did you know that Winston Churchill built one where he wrote some of his famous speeches, and that Queen Victoria also had one where she used to retreat from the pressures of her duties?

If you've never had a place for private thoughts when you were growing up, now is the time to do something about it. Even a single board across a low fork in a sturdy tree fits the fond description 'my tree house', and it's remarkable how much clearer and calmer things seem when you're looking up at the sky through a leafy roof.

If you are lucky enough to have a variety of trees to choose from, select one with low, spreading boughs. This will be easiest to reach when securing a flat, firm and steady platform or floor. Avoid trees such as horse chestnuts or eucalypts, as their limbs tend to snap off under pressure and, naturally, give poisonous shrubs and trees like oleanders a wide berth. The easiest tree house to build is a triangular platform that is secured to the trunk and to two limbs of the tree, resting like a raft on the remaining spreading branches. Clamber up and get away from it all. Sketch, read, think, daydream, eat or just doze for a few minutes … or hours.

52. PLAY DRESS-UPS

Putting on the same clothes in the same way day after relentless day is boring and stifles your creativity. While the solution is not necessarily to go out and spend money on a whole new wardrobe, as every eight-year-old girl knows, you can create a whole new life-story starring yourself just by playing dress-ups ...

Take a fresh look at what you have in your wardrobe. Take out your shirts and tops, scarves and hats, shoes and stockings, and spread them out on the floor or bed. Try different ideas and combinations of clothes and accessories – you are limited only by your imagination.

Don't save a favourite silk scarf for 'best'. Instead, thread it through the belt loops of your jeans and knot it on your hip in a flouncy bow, or tie it to the handle of your tote bag so you can enjoy it every day. Sort through costume jewellery and dress up a beanie or beret with a sparkly over-the-top-dahling diamante brooch. Layer things that you wouldn't usually put together for a spirited, fun, feminine look – try a voile slip dress over a pair of lace tights, then knot a floaty chiffon scarf around your forehead, like a 1920s flapper, or put on red leggings under a big, colourful shirt.

Mix and match office dresses and suits, swapping jackets and skirts to create a different outfit. Even if you wear a uniform to work each day, you can still add a special touch that reflects the real you. Try everything on and strike a pose as you admire your fabulous fashion sense in the mirror!

53. MAKE A BOTTLE GARDEN

A miniature garden growing inside a bottle has the same fascination for us as a ship in a bottle.

Bottle gardens have been used in schools to teach children about the cycles of nature and how all living things are interconnected, and also in rehabilitation hospitals as therapy to improve hand/eye coordination. Making a bottle garden can be as simple or as challenging as you want it to be, providing you with an opportunity for experimentation as well as for moving slowly and carefully, as the plants grow, and developing patience.

Once your bottle garden is established, the plants will grow well, and be protected from draughts, smoke and dust. A bottle garden is a meditation on self-sufficiency. It requires little maintenance as the condensation emitted by the plants is recycled, and the little leaves drop and form mulch, which feeds the next flowering.

BOTTLE GARDEN

a large, flat-based glass bottle, preferably with a wide mouth, (e.g. a wine flagon or large biscuit jar)

small stones or gravel (for the base of the bottle)

sandy soil (you can use potting mix and add sand but make sure it's not too moist or soggy as the plants will rot)

spoon or fork (needs to fit inside the bottle)

a few paddle-pop sticks or short lengths of cane

small plants (e.g. peperomia, begonia, ficus pumila, tradescantia)

cotton reel

◆ Wash and dry the bottle thoroughly. Put stones or gravel in a layer over the base.

◆ Using a funnel, fill the bottle with a layer of dry sandy soil, to between a third and a quarter full.

◆ Tape a spoon to a piece of cane or a paddle-pop stick and use to spread the soil evenly around the bottom of the bottle. Or use a fork taped to a piece of cane as a tiny rake.

◆ With the help of your gardening implements, shape holes and press the plants into the soil. Tamp down the soil using a cotton reel attached to a piece of cane, then water the bottle garden using a fine spray from a pump-mister.

◆ Water the garden infrequently when the plants have settled in as they will be weakened by condensation if they're over watered. Dappled sunlight is best because glass makes the heat too concentrated when the bottle garden is placed in direct sun.

54. BASH A PIÑATA

Why should kids have all the fun? Tearing up lots of strips of newspaper is terrific for getting rid of tension, and making papier-mâché is calming, giving your mind a much-needed break while you use your hands to sculpt and smooth.

Make this piñata for a small friend, or take it into work the next day so you can all take turns to whack it with a ruler to burst the balloon and remove the sweets.

PIÑATA

> old newspapers
> flour
> water
> balloon
> sweets
> paint

◆ Cover a work surface with a few sheets of newspaper. Mix roughly equal quantities of flour and water in a small bucket until you have an opaque, gluey liquid – this is your 'glue'.

◆ Tear up a dozen or so sheets of newspaper into strips about 2.5 cm (1 in) wide.

◆ Blow up the balloon, fill with several handfuls of wrapped sweets, and tie a knot to secure. Sit the balloon in a small bowl so it will stay still while you work. Stir the glue mixture and dip the strips of newspaper in it. Let the excess drip back into the bucket, then stick the strips all over the balloon. Smooth out the strips with your hands. After two or three even layers of newspaper strips have been applied, brush over the shape with a little extra glue and leave the piñata to dry overnight.

◆ When dry, slap on a coat of bright glossy paint. Get creative – perhaps a smiley face or the initials of a friend, if it is to be a present.

55. WRITE A SOAP OPERA

Do you remember playing 'hangman' when you were little? That's the game where you draw a head at the top of a long strip of paper, then fold it out of sight. The next person draws shoulders and folds them out of sight, the next draws a torso, and so on, till you end up with a nonsensical-looking creature.

Get your juices flowing by using the same idea of free association to write a soap opera. This is not only a fun thing to do, it's also a great way of distracting yourself from people or events that are causing you stress. After all, when life is not going to plan, what could be more comforting than to enter a world where you are in control of your characters – what they do and say, and what happens to them – and where things happen precisely as you would like them to do?

Keep a notebook or open a file on your computer, and kick off with the first idea for setting a scene that comes to mind. Where would these take you, for example?

◆ George Georgeson might have been the boss at work, but he wasn't at home. Only last week, the rest of the Georgeson clan …

◆ Just about everyone in the Montville Ladies Auxiliary art class had used the orange scissors this week. How was Detective-Inspector Burrell ever going to identify the killer's prints on the murder weapon?

◆ Laura stretched and yawned and looked out of her window, across to the abandoned lot next door. A movement in the grass caught her eye …

Next time you feel dull and worn out and as though you are just too tired to ever come up with a fresh idea again, take 5 minutes to flick open your 'soapie' script and let your creativity surf in the most surprising directions.

56. MAKE A GRASS 'SCREECHER'

Have you ever whistled on a blade of grass? Besides teaching me how to leap over a tennis net to shake hands with my opponent (my game was dreadful, but my good sportsmanship was impressive) and how to make a perfect pink gin, my father taught me how to make grass 'screechers'.

Making a screecher is one of the more satisfying stress-busters I've found, making an ear-splitting 'alley-oop!' type of whistle and relaxing your jaw to boot. I have yet to perfect the ability to play a tune on one, though Edward does this effortlessly.

Pick a piece of grass – as wide and firm as possible – and make a slit in it with your thumbnail. Hold it between your thumb and first finger on each hand over your pursed lips. Pull it tight, hold on to the edges, and then blow.

57. DECORATE EGGS

What is it about the smooth, even shape of an egg that is so calming and soothing? Perhaps it's because they're a traditional symbol of rebirth and new beginnings.

Decorated eggs are probably best known as a traditional Easter craft, but they can also be used to make an appealing collection of personal mementoes of important events. Display them in a bowl and they will bring back positive memories each time you pass by.

Decorating eggs is an opportunity for creative expression. However, unlike many hobbies, there is no opportunity for competition – whatever you do is purely for the pleasure of it. Let your intuition and emotions decide what will be the subject. Remember that the impact of this craft lies in the fact that you have to focus on just one simple message or symbol: something that's small enough to fit on an egg, such as a little brown teddy on a pale blue egg to mark the birth of a baby boy, or a tiny red aeroplane and a palm tree to signify an overseas holiday.

Decorated Eggs

eggs
egg cups
fine paintbrush
paint, glitter, beads, as desired
clear varnish

◆ Pierce the pointed end of an egg with a needle, then make a slightly larger hole in the flatter end. Let the white and yolk run out into a bowl, rinse the shell carefully and allow it to dry. You can make this happen a bit faster by blowing into the small hole, forcing the contents out of the large hole into the bowl.

◆ Stand each blown egg in an egg cup and decorate as desired. Carefully paint all over the egg with the clear varnish and leave to dry completely.

58. PLAY HAND SHADOWS

This isn't just a kids' game. Like most meaningful meditative practices, it takes you outside of your busy brain for a few moments, helps you loosen up and relax, and restores perspective.

All you need is a light and a blank section of wall. Close the curtains or blinds if necessary. Hold your hands a metre or so from the wall and adjust them till the shadow looks sharp.

My dad taught me how to make this shadow dog.

♦ Press both palms together, keeping the first three fingers of both hands together and moving the two little fingers back towards your arm together – this makes the dog's mouth, which you can open and shut.

♦ To make the ears, separate your thumbs.

♦ If circumstances permit, say 'Roaaaarr! Sic 'em, buddy', make growling noises, and watch your pup attack your imagined problems and send them packing, tails between their legs.

59. MAKE FLOWER HONEY

There are many creative ways of using flowers to add colour and romance to your life besides arranging them in a vase. Not only do flowers look and smell sweet, many taste delightful, too. Apple blossom, elderflowers, honeysuckle, rose petals and lavender are just a few of the flowers that can be used to add flavour and colour to food. Herbs such as mint and lemon balm work well too.

Use a good quality, organic honey for best results. Commercially prepared honeys don't taste as good. Do not use flowers that have been sprayed with pesticides or herbicides.

Flower Honey

> 1 cup fragrant flower petals, lightly bruised
> 500 g (16 oz) clear organic honey

◆ Place the flower petals in a clean glass jar and pour over the warmed honey. Leave the jar in a warm, sunny place for 10 days or longer, until the honey takes on the delicate taste and scent of the flowers. Strain and rebottle.

60. CREATE A SIGNATURE SCENT

People seem to be experiencing more irritation from – if not allergies to – the synthetic chemicals that permeate twenty-first century life. For a more personal, sexier effect, try creating your own fragrance from fresh flowers – it's fun and relaxing to play at being a modern-day apothecary.

ROSE PERFUME

> 1 cup rose petals (dark red are best – they have the strongest perfume)
> 1 cup vodka
> 2 cups boiling water
> clingwrap
> 2 tablespoons fresh rosemary, chopped
> 2 tablespoons grated orange zest

◆ Place the rose petals in a china bowl and bruise with a wooden spoon or pestle. Add ½ cup of the vodka and mix well. Pour over 1 cup of boiling water. Cover the bowl with clingwrap and store in a cool, dry place for 10 days.

◆ Place the rosemary and orange zest in a bowl and bruise with a wooden spoon or pestle. Add the remaining vodka and boiling water, cover with clingwrap and set aside for 10 days.

◆ After 10 days, strain off the rose petals and rosemary–orange mixture. Strain a second time through a coffee filter to remove the grit. Combine the two and store in a clean, dark-coloured glass bottle. Shake well before use.

61. GO HIPPIE

Tie-dyeing was hugely popular during the 1970s – the combination of creating unstructured, random designs, slowly stirring pots of brightly coloured dye, and giving an old T-shirt or a pair of pillowslips a new lease of life is liberating, relaxing and satisfying all at once. It is also an inexpensive, hands-on opportunity to see something old, familiar – even boring – in a new light, and to transform it into something new and exciting that you can use almost straightaway. Maybe it's time to bring the practice back!

There is the creative satisfaction that you get from working with colour and pattern. It's a great craft to try if you are feeling stuck or worn-out.

Tie-dyed Fabrics

    cold-water fabric dye
    old white T-shirts or sheets
    rubber bands

- ◆ Make up the dye in a bucket according to the manufacturer's instructions.

- ◆ Roll up or pleat the material. Wind the rubber bands tightly around the fabric at intervals – this will create wiggly whitish strips, because the dye won't be able to get to the fabric in those places.

- ◆ Put on rubber gloves. Place the item in the bucket of dye, stirring gently with a stick or old wooden spoon.

- ◆ Still with the rubber gloves on, lift the item into the sink and rinse according to the manufacturer's instructions (usually one rinse in hot water, then a second in cold).

- ◆ Leave the wet item on a pile of old newspapers to dry. When dry, cut away the rubber bands.

62. MAKE CANDLES

Gaze into a candle flame and you are at once connected to the past and to the future. It manages to convey energy, comfort and hope all at once. Consider the rich words of this ancient prayer, older than time, which is still recited at the Jewish Feast of Lights when the candles are lit: 'May this candle's radiance pour upon our hearts and spread light into the darkened corners of the world.'

There's something very soothing and satisfying about working with the texture of wax, and polishing its smooth surface. And making them is child's play. There's an old tradition in Spain that says a candle should be lit and placed on the windowsill so the Christ child can find his way on Christmas Eve, but you don't have to wait for Christmas to make your window come alive each evening. Make a candle – or a group of them – and arrange them on a windowsill to show a friendly light to passers-by.

CANDLES

> candle moulds and wicks (from craft shop)
> 350 g (12 oz) paraffin wax
> 35 g (1 oz) stearin (from craft shop – makes candles harden, and more opaque)
> essential oil
> cottonwool
> vegetable oil

♦ Lightly coat moulds with vegetable oil and insert wicks following the manufacturer's instructions. (There are usually six moulds in a set, depending on the size and shape of the candle you want.) You can also recycle milk cartons and cut away at the end.

♦ Melt the wax in the top half of an old double-boiler over simmering water. Melt the stearin in another old, small saucepan, then add to the wax and stir. Add the essential oil now if you wish to include it.

♦ Pour the wax into the moulds and allow to set. When the candles are firm, trim the wicks. To give the candles a smooth finish, polish them with cottonwool dipped in vegetable oil.

63. PUT ON LIPSTICK

The simplest, most commonplace actions often have the most restorative and empowering effects.

Perhaps it's my mother's influence (she would no more leave the house in the morning without wearing lipstick than she would go out without wearing knickers), but I find that whipping out a lipstick and applying it is a quick pick-me-up that rarely fails. In just a few seconds, I look better, feel brighter, more confident, and I know I am more optimistic, and more able to deal with things when I have – as Randall describes it – 'coloured in my face'. That creative little touch of colour is a private signal to my inner self, a private rosy proof that I can reclaim time to do something that is utterly, selfishly and completely for my benefit.

64. GO FLY A KITE

'I saw you toss a kite on high, and blow the birds about the sky,' wrote Robert Louis Stevenson in A Child's Garden of Verses.

His words sum up the romance and sense of freedom that comes with flying a kite – you're connected with the darting birds and gusting clouds up there by just a piece of string.

Kite-flying is a great stress-buster – dashing back and forth at the park or wherever you are, just trying to keep that kite aloft, pushes your cares away to the back of your mind. Fill your lungs with fresh air and watch your kite soar upwards, lifting your spirits with it.

You can buy a very inexpensive kite from a toy store, or make your own as an easy, fun craft project.

KITE

crepe paper
2 pieces of light dowelling, one 40 cm (16 in) long, one 60 cm (2 ft) long
nails
4 small eyelet screws
string
firm paper
craft glue
cardboard
long piece of twine
cardboard

◆ Cut a tail and tassels for the kite from the crepe paper.

◆ Place the shorter piece of dowelling over the longer one about a third of the way down to form a cross shape. Tack the pieces together.

◆ Twist a tiny eyelet screw into each of the four ends of the dowelling. Run a length of string through the four eye holes and tie to form a diamond shape.

◆ Spread the firm paper flat on the floor and place the wooden frame on top. Trace the outline of the string with a pen. Add another 10 cm (4 in) around all four sides and cut out the shape. Glue the edges, turning them over the string all the way around. Attach the tail and tassels at each end of the crosswise strip.

◆ Thread a piece of string through each of the eyelet holes. Knot the pieces together in the centre back of the kite; the knot should be about 45 cm (18 in) out from the frame and at right angles to the intersection of the pieces of dowelling.

◆ Make a spool out of cardboard. Wind the long twine over it. Tie the end of the twine to the knot in the centre of the kite.

65. PLAY IN THE SAND

Spending any time at all near the ocean restores perspective and puts roses back in your cheeks. Walking along the wet sand puts you in touch with nature. See how the waterline changes as the tide flows in and out, gaze at the horizon and feel the tangy breeze on your cheeks.

Playing in the sand is not just for children – hunkering down and getting sand between your toes (and in your hair, on your salty lips, and inside your swimmers) is one of the most satisfying and relaxing stress-busters you'll find. Try these sandy time-out ideas.

◆ Bury a friend in sand up to the neck. Shape the sand around their body into a rocket or a racing car.

◆ Right at the edge of the sea, where the sand is wet, build an enormous turtle or monster coming out of the sea. Mark out its eyes and fins with shells and seaweed.

◆ Build a sand mountain of damp sand. Deliberately and gleefully leap on top of it, and destroy your creation. Shout: 'I'm the king of the castle, and you're the dirty rascal!' Who cares? No need to feel remorse – know that there will be more days ahead, more sand mountains and more chances to celebrate the joy of being alive.

◆ Take a stick and draw a giant circle in the sand. Inside the circle, write the name of a person who's giving you grief, or draw a picture of something that's bothering you – a stick figure of your boss, perhaps, or a dollar sign for money, a broken heart for a relationship problem. Sit in your circle with your symbol for a few moments, then get up and step out again. Walk away, leaving your problem inside the circle. Soon, your drawing will be washed away, a process that represents the transience of existence and the cycle of life, and your problem will have disappeared with it.

66. BAKE GINGERBREAD

What is it about the mouth-wateringly spicy scent of gingerbread that makes us shut our eyes and feel all warm and toasty, right down to our toes?

Decorate with icing or chocolate drops or tiny coloured choc buttons and take them into work as a treat for colleagues tomorrow – if they last that long.

GINGERBREAD

4 tablespoons butter
2 cups brown sugar
2 eggs, well beaten
2 tablespoons milk
4 tablespoons golden syrup
2 teaspoons bicarbonate of soda
4 cups plain (all-purpose) flour
2 teaspoons ground cinnamon
3 teaspoons ground ginger
1 teaspoon cream of tartar

- Preheat the oven to 200°C (400°F). Grease baking sheets with butter and line with baking paper.

- Cream the butter and sugar. Add the eggs and beat until the mixture is creamy.

- Combine the milk, golden syrup and bicarbonate of soda and add to the egg mixture. Mix until combined.

- Sift the flour, cinnamon, ginger and cream of tartar together and stir into the mixture, mixing very well.

- Shape the dough into a rectangle and roll out on a well-floured board to 1 cm (½ in) thickness. Using decorative cutters – hearts, stars and crescent moons all look good – cut out shapes.

- Place on the baking sheets and cook for 20–30 minutes. Do not allow them to brown. Let the biscuits cool on racks. They will be softish when they come out of the oven and firm up as they cool.

REMEMBER TO RELAX AND TAKE TIME OUT TO **CREATE** ...

67. INVENT A HOLIDAY

What a wonderful, calming and inspirational word 'holiday' is – you only have to say it, and you can feel yourself start to unwind and smile with anticipation. But we get so few of them! And – unfortunately – official holidays such as Christmas are marked by time constraints and too-high expectations that can result in a stressful jumble of driving, shopping, packing and duty-calls visits to relatives.

Why not invent a holiday each month, or find an unusual or forgotten one to celebrate? Here are some from other countries and religions.

◆ **Onam** is celebrated as a harvest festival in India during the first week of August. Traditionally, people dress up in new clothes and decorate their homes with beautiful flower arrangements.

◆ **Guy Fawkes Day** is celebrated on 5 November; in England, the celebrations feature fireworks and bonfires.

◆ **Thanksgiving** was first celebrated in America by the pilgrim fathers to mark their gratitude for a good harvest.

Celebrate anniversaries of personal achievements, your own and other people's. Observe birthdays of famous people – my husband Doug always celebrates Shakespeare's birthday on 23 April with candles, nice food and a toast to the Bard.

Mark the first day of spring by wearing a sprig of blossom in your jacket lapel, or make a big bowl of mango sorbet on the first day of summer. As well as adding a bit of fun and excitement to life, the great thing about inventing holidays is that you don't actually have to take time off work if you're not able to do so. What it does is change your attitude towards the day – it's no longer another ordinary day, it's a special one.

68. WEAVE A LAVENDER WAND

Here's a fun craft idea to try. As a bonus, the sweet scent of lavender has a settling effect on nerves and will soothe a tension headache. Once you get the hang of it, you can make one of these wands in just minutes. And it doesn't matter if you have two left thumbs – if you can plait hair, you can make these.

LAVENDER WAND

> 12 fresh lavender flowers, on stems as long as possible
> narrow pink or mauve ribbon, about 1 metre (39 in) long

◆ Using the ribbon, tie the lavender flowers together firmly just beneath the flower heads.

◆ Bend each of the stems back gently below the ribbon so that they form a 'cage' over the flowers, and then tie the bottom of the stems together. Be gentle, though if you use fresh lavender the stems are pliable and won't catch or break.

◆ Weave the long ends of the ribbon over and under the stems, moving down the wand until all the lavender is enclosed. Maintain tension so you have a snug and neat wand. Stitch the ribbon ends together firmly, and finish with a bow.

69. MAKE MARMALADE

The very word 'marmalade' is soothing to say out loud – all those ms, and that sweet, poetic rhythm. Making preserves like marmalade is one of those quietly restorative tasks that puts you in touch with simpler times.

As you chop and peel and mix and taste, think of the generations of women before you who have stirred pots of spicy fruit, waiting for the precise moment when their mixture would gel, and breathing in the clean, sweet, homey fragrance all the while. There's also something very satisfying about seeing all the jars neatly lined up on shelves. I like to sneak a peek and admire my hard work, then shut the pantry door again, knowing that there are many months' worth of enjoyment to be had.

Select only smooth, thin-skinned oranges. Fruit is best when there is next to no thickening of the rind at either blossom or stem end. If this thickening is present, cut off a slice from either end to prevent bitterness.

Whisky Marmalade

1 kg (2 lb) firm, ripe, thin-skinned oranges
250 g (8 oz) glacé ginger, finely chopped
3 tablespoons ground ginger
6 tablespoons whisky
caster sugar

◆ Wash the oranges thoroughly. Peel the fruit with a vegetable peeler. Cut the peel into long fine strips, reserving the pith. Cut the fruit into chunks and place with the peel in a large non-aluminium saucepan. Remove and save any seeds.

◆ Place the pith and seeds in a muslin bag, tie securely and place in the saucepan with the fruit peel, both gingers and whisky. Add enough water to barely cover, place the lid on the saucepan and leave to soak overnight.

◆ Bring the mixture to the boil and simmer until the peel is tender. Reduce the heat to low and cook until mixture is pulpy – about 40 minutes. Stir regularly to make sure it's not sticking to the bottom of the pan. Discard the muslin bag.

◆ Measure the pulp and add 1 cup of sugar for every cup of pulp. Bring to the boil to dissolve the sugar and cook until the setting point is reached. Test this by spooning a little jam onto a plate and chilling it in the fridge. If the cooled jam wrinkles when you push it with your finger, it has reached setting point. Spoon into sterile glass jars and cap securely.

70. A STITCH IN TIME

We all face that relentless round of cooking and cleaning every week. The frustration inherent in most domestic duties is that you have nothing to show for them – you wake up the next day, and the laundry basket is overflowing again, and more dirty dishes are stacked up in the sink. No trace of your time and hard work survives.

Needlework, however, lasts. For centuries, all styles of sewing have provided women with a creative outlet, and borne testimony to their preoccupations, beliefs and values. It is fascinating to walk through exhibits of handcrafted rag dolls and embroidered baby clothes at country fairs or to sift through piles of folded soft patchwork quilts and pillowslips trimmed with drawn threadwork and cross-stitch in old wares stores. While the way of life of women and girls who dreamed of a world beyond their front gates may have gone, the lesson of sitting and methodically stitching away remains a valuable one in today's stressed-out world.

Embroidery is a simple and effective way to restore perspective at the end of the day, absorbing your mind and giving you a great feeling of satisfaction. Simple needlework kits are available in craft and department stores. Settle yourself in a comfortable chair with plenty of natural light, thread the needle with the coloured silk or wool, and start.

A fragrant pillow will delicately perfume your bedroom, help to calm your nerves and induce a restful, deep sleep. Use your hands to blend the dried flowers and herbs; enjoy the feel of the crisp, dried petals between your fingertips, and breathe in the clean, soft fragrance. This handkerchief pillow is easily made by sewing two lace-edged handkerchiefs together, with the trim outermost. No sewing machine? Just hand-sew around the three sides, using small, straight stitches, and enjoy watching the needle moving easily in and out.

Sleep Pillow

3 tablespoons dried lavender
1 tablespoon dried chamomile
1 teaspoon dried marjoram
lavender essential oil
handkerchief case

◆ Gently crush the dried herbs and flowers together in a bowl, mixing thoroughly. Stir in 5 drops of the essential oil. (Add a few drops of brandy to help fix and strengthen the scent.)

◆ Pour the mixture into the handkerchief case, then turn in the ends of the open seam and sew up.

◆ Tuck the pillow between your usual pillow and pillowcase, so it will release its scent whenever you rest on it.

71. READ – OR WRITE – A POEM

The right poem at the right time can be the perfect answer when you're feeling frightened, confused or just plain irritated. No matter how bad things look, chances are some poet has been there before you, and has encapsulated your thoughts and feelings in just a few insightful words.

Need courage? Be inspired by the stirring words of Rudyard Kipling's 'If' ('If you can keep your head when all about you are losing theirs'). Had your heart broken? Look up anything by Dorothy Parker and feel the beginnings of a wry smile. Centuries-old Japanese haiku can be incredibly evocative; the very economy of words communicates serenity. Try reading your chosen poem aloud: researchers have found that this helps to relax and synchronise your heart and breathing rates more than if you read in your head.

Writing poetry is also a blissful secret release for tension and pent-up emotions. No special training is required. Get a pen and paper, or open a blank file on your computer. Close your eyes and think of the person or situation that is on your mind. This could be a positive or a negative experience or emotion, or perhaps something to do with work, or even your unexpressed feelings about an old lover or a difficult child. Describe in a few words how you feel about that person or situation. If you can't come up with the right words, describe your emotions by likening your feelings to images. For example:

♦ I feel as though there is a disco ball hanging over my head, throwing light in every direction. Which way do I turn?

♦ You make me feel so happy when I see you; to know that you care what happens fills me with energy. I feel as though I am plugged in to a power point!

♦ I feel like a caterpillar in its cocoon – I can see the light outside, but I need to break through what's holding me back so I can grow and spread my wings.

Not all of your poems will be easy or positive. But writing poetry can be a shortcut to accurately identifying sources of frustration and anger so you can deal with them. Rather than wallowing in emotions and writing for pages and pages, really concentrate on a few descriptive phrases that sum up your feelings to help you examine the essence of an experience.

72. DECORATE YOUR LETTERBOX

When my friend Pat lived on a farm she was known to kids for miles around as 'the letterbox lady'. What they were referring to was Pat's habit of decorating her letterbox in all sorts of surprising ways, as the mood took her. Sometimes she tied on a bunch of flowers; other days, it was balloons. One Christmas, she decked it with red and green baubles and set a small tree on top, complete with winking lights. During football season, she draped it with scarves and flags. When her prize mare's long-awaited filly arrived after several days of agonised waiting, she propped a sign against the box saying 'It's a girl!' One Easter she set up a giant grey rabbit carrying a big basket of eggs – the word got around so fast that the school bus was asked to make a detour so the kids could go and collect their eggs!

Pat is still coming up with ideas for decorating her letterbox. It has become a talking point in her community – tourists knock on her door and ask her permission to take photos, and the local newspaper even interviewed her. When the journalist asked her why she did it, she quoted that wonderful, inspiring line from Robert F. Kennedy: 'Some dream of things that are, and say "Why?" I dream of things that never were and say, "Why not?"'

A mailbox with an ever-changing message? Why not, indeed? Decorate your letterbox with a plaster gnome or a teddy bear, trim a tree or shrubs in your front garden with fairy lights or tinsel, hang a string of bells from a gate-post, and send out a positive signal into the universe. You'll lift your mood knowing that passers-by will see it and be surprised into a smile.

73. MAKE A DEN

When my sons were small, they loved to make camps and forts: elaborate, tent-like tunnels and structures out of old cardboard boxes, pieces of wood and throw-rugs, all stretched between chairs and under tables. They would crawl in one end with some cushions, a torch, some toys and illicit supplies of food and drink, and they'd be happy for hours.

Everyone needs a den, a safe, cosy haven where you can hide from the world, no matter how old you are. Making your home a warm, welcoming place is important, but the idea of creating a private space that's just for you takes it one step further. Your den can be as large or as small as you like. If you have a large home, you may be able to set aside a whole room just for you to retreat to, and furnish it with a favourite armchair, ceiling-high shelves of books, a sewing table or a workbench for craft. You might even be able to indulge dreams of converting an attic or cellar, of building a loft room over a garage, or building a garden summerhouse. One of my friends has rescued an old red painted telephone booth and has plans for turning it into a tiny sitting-room-for-one in a sunny corner of her garden.

Even if you're really pushed for space, you can still drape a curtain across a corner of a room to create a private spot with a pile of cushions, or put a chair next to a window with a small table on which to place a cup. The smallest and simplest spot has the potential to be a tranquil, restorative place, a still-point in your life that gives you the chance for a refreshing break, or a little reflection, helping to restore your physical and emotional balance.

Use the following suggestions to make a den that will replenish your body and soul. Don't go overboard – we all have so much stimulation in our lives that just carving out one still corner will be a tonic.

◆ **Set your den apart with some sort of buffer** If not a door, then a length of voile, or a row of potted plants. Make an entrance. A bead curtain or a chain of bells can denote an entry at which cares can be left behind.

◆ **Have a focal point** Artist Paul Klee wrote, 'We have two eyes – one to see, the other to feel'. Inspire one eye with something beautiful – a vase of flowers, a collection of distinctively marked shells or pebbles, or a painting. Then feed the other eye – your 'feeling' eye – with something from nature or another ethnic culture that has spiritual or cultural significance. A beautiful woven wall-hanging or a hand-carved wooden bowl feeds the spirit as well as your aesthetic sense, and reminds you that people everywhere are intrinsically good and creative. Some of them have nothing, yet they create the most extraordinary things.

◆ **A place to sit – or lie down – is crucial** Find a comfortable chair, a beanbag or pile of cushions, or an old-fashioned chaise longue or Balinese day-bed.

◆ **Choose colours that please you** Deep rich purples, pale blue and white are best for a restful feel. Scent also enhances the ambience of your den – light vanilla or lavender incense to calm you down, or place an aromatherapy diffuser nearby.

74. ASSEMBLE A MODEL

When I was little, rainy days would see me totally absorbed in making my latest model kit doll's house. I raised walls, glued banisters to stairwells, built fences and laid tiles, then painted window ledges, gutters and down pipes. I pieced together tiny tables and chairs and varnished them, framed postage stamps with toothpicks to make portraits to hang. Making these models not only kept me out of my mother's hair for hours on end, it was one of the happiest and most contented times of my life.

Adults can also benefit from this hobby. It's absorbing, which helps you to relax, and there's also something symbolic about making anything in miniature, whether it's a house, a plane or a boat. Perhaps it's the sense of escaping into another world, one where you have complete control over what happens, even if your waking world is unpredictable.

Model-making teaches you patience, and forces you to be methodical and to take a slow and steady approach. Take the time to ponder: each little piece needs to be found, placed in just the right position, glued and allowed to dry before you proceed to the next step. If you try to take shortcuts, or you're not paying attention, the model won't turn out properly and your work will be wasted. In many ways, model-making is a metaphor for life – patiently waiting to see patterns develop and then, when the time is right, being decisive and taking action.

Visit your craft or toy shop and choose a model kit – an easy one to start with, to develop your skills and build your confidence. It's satisfying to work with your hands and to see your model develop a tiny little bit at a time.

75. SEW A PERUVIAN WORRY DOLL

These powerful lucky charms originated many centuries ago. It is still traditional for Peruvian mothers to tuck one into their child's bedding or to hang one on a string around their neck. The doll is supposed to capture dangerous spirits and put them in the bag at her waist, then draw the string tight so they cannot escape. In the morning, the mother would open the bag and shoo them away. It's not just small children who can feel comforted by this idea – if you're feeling stressed or besieged by bad luck you could pop a Peruvian worry doll under your pillow, just to be on the safe side.

Peruvian Worry Doll

>   fabric
>   thread, yarn, cottonwool
>   tiny buttons or beads, wool, marker pens

◆ Cut out a piece of fabric about 6.5 cm x 9 cm (2½ x 3½ in). Fold in half lengthwise and oversew the long side and one short side. Turn inside out. Fill with cottonwool, then sew up remaining short side.

◆ Tie a length of coloured yarn about a quarter of the way down to form the head. Cut a semicircle of fabric and glue or stitch in place around the doll's neck to form her cape. Now decorate her face and hair by gluing on buttons and lengths of wool or using marker pens to make a face and hair. Decorate the cape by gluing on fabric scraps, beads or feathers.

◆ Cut out a circle of fabric and run a drawstring thread around the outside; pull it up to make a bag, and tie it to the doll's waist.

76. GROW A RAINBOW GARDEN

Rainbows are one of the most beautiful sights in nature. One moment the sky is heavy with rain and in the next instant, a gigantic arch with bands of sparkling colour is soaring overhead. No wonder the ancient Greeks believed the goddess Iris lived in rainbows, and no wonder we search for pots of gold at their end.

Keep that sense of romance and playful, childlike wonder alive by growing your own rainbow. Gardening in any form is relaxing because it's good exercise, and the repetitive act of weeding, digging or planting out seedlings is almost like a peaceful meditation.

Your rainbow garden can be as small or as large as you like. Mark out strips in a window box or a flowerbed, then plant out every strip in flowers or foliage to match the colours of the rainbow. For example, you might have a strip of red hot pokers, then one of yellow marigolds, purple pansies, blue forget-me-nots, pink alyssum, and so on. Annuals such as hot pink portulaca and blue lobelia will survive an amateur scatter-planting on a larger scale, and grow practically anywhere. Orange or yellow nasturtiums quickly germinate to form a colourful display.

When your rainbow garden is in its glory, take a colour photo and pin it to your bulletin board or put it on your fridge door. Every time you see it, you will be cheered and inspired by this pretty reminder of nature's bounty.

77. MAKE A BATCH OF SCONES

Most of the actions associated with cooking – the stirring, the mixing, the spooning – are soothing and rewarding, and provide the cook with an opportunity to slow down and savour the moment, to say nothing about the privileges of licking the spoon! And nothing says 'welcome' like freshly baked scones. They're easy to make, and they're ready in minutes. As a bonus, the kneading of the dough is a great way to thump out some stress. Break one open while it's still hot, spread with whipped cream and strawberry jam and then take a bite …

SCONES

½ teaspoon vegetable oil
200 g (1⅓ cups) self-raising flour
50 g (½ stick) butter, cubed
grated zest of 1 orange
50 g (2 oz) dried apricots, finely chopped (optional)
3 teaspoons sugar
60 ml (¼ cup) buttermilk
1 tablespoon sour cream

◆ Preheat the oven to 220°C (425°F). Lightly grease a baking sheet with the oil, and set aside.

◆ Sift the flour into a bowl and rub in the butter until the mixture is crumbly. Add the zest, apricots and sugar, then mix in the buttermilk and sour cream to form a workable dough.

◆ Turn out onto a lightly floured surface and knead until smooth.

◆ Roll out the dough to a thickness of 2.5 cm (1 in) and cut out rounds using a pastry cutter.

◆ Place on baking sheet, leaving plenty of space between. Brush with extra buttermilk, pop in the oven and cook for 8–10 minutes, or until the tops are brown.

78. WORK ON A JIGSAW

One of the sweetest memories I have of Randall when he was small is of us working on an absolutely enormous jigsaw puzzle together. It was a scene of a pine forest and contained over 1000 pieces no larger than a thumbnail, nearly all of which were green. We spread the pieces out on the floor and whiled away many pleasant, quiet hours, first putting together the outline, then filling in the middle, bit by bit. And woe betide anyone who moved anything!

The reason that jigsaws are so relaxing is that your mind is completely absorbed by the task of finding the next right-shaped piece. Unlike other games such as playing chess or cards, there is no need to think about options or strategies, or to remember what someone's last move or bid was. You can play it alone or with a partner, without any sense of competition. Unlike most hobbies or pastimes, you can simply get up and do something else if you have to, without having to worry about packing up and putting things away, or getting stressed about leaving at a critical time. Whether you've just begun, or you've almost finished, 'jigsaw time' is all the same: there is no sense of having to hurry up, or of not being able to leave in case you miss something or forget your place or lose your momentum.

Two tips, though. One: don't make the mistake that Ran and I made of tackling such a huge jigsaw. Pick one that has between 100 and 200 pieces to begin with, so that you won't be discouraged. And choose a picture with a lot of contrasting colours.

79. HAVE A PERSONAL LUCKY CHARM

I have two lucky charms, a four-leafed clover encased in a tiny plastic sleeve and a St Christopher medallion, both of which I keep in my wallet. I have never been to Ireland, and I rarely travel, but I feel more comfortable knowing that they are there. Every so often I will touch them, just to be on the safe side.

Lucky charms are as old as humankind. Perhaps the need for supernatural protection is hardwired into us, harking back to days of wizards, witch doctors and high priestesses, talking trees, swords in stones and amulets with supernatural powers. Perhaps it's just a childish need for security and reassurance, or the sweet knowledge of having a secret about which no one else knows.

A lucky charm can be anything – a smooth stone, a toy truck, a cross, a tiny Buddha, a feather, a champagne cork or a vial of coloured sand. A quick survey of friends reveals a rabbit's foot, a broken hat pin, an eagle's feather, a shell, a thimble, a silver earring, a piece of agate, a baby bracelet and an Armed Forces pin from an Australian digger's slouch hat.

These lucky charms have two things in common. One, each has a special story, and each came into that person's life at a significant time, or reminds them of a certain person or occasion, or of characteristics or values they want to keep with them. And two, they are all small, meaning they can be easily carried about.

Perhaps you already have a lucky charm? There may be a personal item you use every day, like a pendant or a key ring, something that you like to touch occasionally, something you don't feel quite right going out into the world without. Next time you feel overwhelmed, hold your lucky charm tightly and take several deep breaths. Notice your conscious mind come back into focus, your breathing become more relaxed. Your day is back on an even keel.

80. MAKE A WREATH

Wreaths are very pleasing to look at, as well as being objects of great symbolic significance. Our ancestors regarded the perfect circle as a powerful device that brought harmony and good fortune; the circle was thought in many cultures to ward off the evil eye, which explains the origins of the traditional Christmas wreath.

Creating a wreath is physically calming and emotionally soothing. When you sit and work with your hands, you cannot help but feel more settled and grounded, and using treasures from nature like dried moss and scented pine cones shift your thoughts towards the natural world. The circular form of the wreath is also a subtle visual prompt towards relaxation as you work your way around, tucking in sweet-smelling cinnamon sticks, gluing on nuts or tying on bows. See your work as part of the circle of life.

Wreath

> cane, vine or wire ring base from a craft shop
> florist moss
> decorative materials: your choice of fresh or dried herbs, flowers and grasses (e.g. hydrangea, gypsophila, chamomile, dried ferns, miniature lotus pods, poppyseed cases, rosemary sprigs); fruit (e.g. cumquats and pomegranates, small oranges studded with cloves); spices (e.g. cinnamon sticks, vanilla pods, whole nutmegs or walnuts, star anise, bay leaves); nuts (e.g. pine cones, chestnuts and other unshelled nuts); small balls or beads
> glue
> satin ribbon

◆ Pad the ring base with florist moss to disguise it.

◆ Starting at one side and working in one direction, tuck in the spices, flowers, nuts and herbs, adding a dab of clear craft glue if necessary to secure. Overlap to conceal any stems and ends you want to keep hidden.

◆ Finish the wreath by gluing or tying a loop of satin ribbon to the top of the wreath to use for hanging. If the wreath is particularly heavy, attach a wire loop to the back of the wreath at the top, where it can't be seen. Try misting the wreath with an essential oil such as rosemary diluted in a little vodka to give it a long-lasting fragrance.

81. LOOK THROUGH A LENS

My son Edward took up photography at school this year and he has produced quirky collages made up of the faces, hands, shoes, eyes and ears of his friends and teachers. The message he's trying to put across is that we're all different, yet all the same; all connected, yet separate. He enjoys photography so much he has even said he'd like to be a photographer when he grows up.

'Why photography?' I asked.

'Because it makes you get closer and really notice things, and you can also change the way things go together,' he answered.

How you see the world depends on your mood, your attitude and your habits. If you're used to seeing things in a certain way, you can become rigid in your thinking, and stuck in your ways. Photography is not just a relaxing hobby or even an opportunity for creative expression; it can be a way of making you see the world through fresh eyes. When you look through a camera lens, even just for a few moments, you are taking the time to really appreciate what you are seeing because you are focusing on the details – shadows passing over a church spire, a child's gap-toothed smile, the way your daughter's hair falls so sweetly over her forehead, the brilliant greens and reds in a bunch of fresh radishes. Later, you can do as Ed has done and actually manipulate those images – create a whole new reality – by playing with technology and adjusting colours, shapes and sizes, and so make an intensely personal statement.

Looking at the world through a lens can change your perception of what is around you, alerting you to what is beautiful and inspiring in plain view that you would otherwise walk past. You don't have to buy an expensive camera – just pick up a disposable one at the chemist and take it with you to the park. Hold it up and, as you look through it, see the ordinary world around you become extraordinary. Notice kids on scooters, unexpected flowers, the three rusty bikes that are parked in a line, branches overhead with blue sky beyond, a beautiful cloud.

82. SMASH SOME CHINA

My friend Jane is one of the calmest, sanest and most well-balanced people I have ever met. She smells of White Linen, her cuticles are always pushed back, and she is so warm and relaxed she could make the North Pole seem comfy with just a couple of deckchairs and a candle. Her secret?

'Tuesday nights,' she says. 'That's my mosaic class. I wouldn't miss it.'

Making mosaics is fail-safe stress relief. However bad a mood you're in to start with, you can be assured of feeling better when you've finished. It's easy and inexpensive – no training is required, and you need very little equipment. It's creatively satisfying, because you end up producing something useful and attractive, and it may just save your sanity. Far better to take out your pent-up aggression on old cups and saucers than on the exasperating Ms Perkins from the Accounts department.

Most local community colleges and art centres offer courses in mosaic-making that you can sign up for. Or it's quite easy to do it yourself at home.

Mosaic

old blanket or rug
selection of old or chipped cups and odd plates, preferably with a colourful
design or pattern
piece of heavy particleboard, about 30 cm (12 in) square
craft or china glue
tube of ready-made grouting
eyelet screws and wire or rope

◆ Spread the blanket or rug on grass or over an old thick mat on a patio or terrace. Place the china in the centre and fold in the ends several times so that there are no openings where pieces can fly out.

◆ Put on gardening gloves and protective glasses and smash the china with a meat mallet or hammer. Unwrap the rug or blanket and carefully pick over the pieces. Wrap any that are still too big back in the blanket and bash them again till they're all around the same size. Repeat until all the china pieces are roughly the same size, about 2.5 cm (1 in) square and flattish.

◆ Spread the pieces out on a sheet of paper and play with them until you have a design that you like. A simple graphic image, such as a star or a fish or a spiral, will work well.

◆ Place the particleboard next to the sheet of paper. Using craft or china glue, pick up each piece of china from the paper with your fingers or tweezers, glue the back, and stick it onto the board.

◆ To finish, squeeze grouting around all the pieces to secure the mosaic and give it an even surface. Sponge or wipe off any excess according to the manufacturer's instructions.

◆ When the grouting is thoroughly dry, screw in the eyelets about 5 cm (2 in) from the top and thread a length of wire or rope between them to hang the work.

83. KEEP A BUTTON BOX

Growing up in my grandmother's house, I would spend rainy afternoons playing with a box filled with odd buttons and beads. Sometimes I would string them onto lengths of wool or cotton to make an endless variety of necklaces and bracelets. But most of all, I would just pick up handfuls and then pour them back into the box, like a clattering waterfall. I never realised how deeply satisfying and comforting this was until I came across a button box in an antique shop. It was filled to the brim with all sorts of buttons – round, square, pearl, silver, toggle, glittery, painted, wooden and plain. Straightaway I dipped in and scooped up a handful, then let them run through my fingers. I bought the box and took it home.

Keep a collection of buttons or small beads or pebbles in a small bowl or box. Put it on an occasional table or a bureau near a lamp so that soft light falls on them in the evening. Play with them each time you pass.

84. DESIGN A ZEN GARDEN

Amanda is godmother to my sons, and she is famous for giving them thoughtful and unusual gifts. This year, she gave Randall a kit to make a miniature Zen garden, modelled on the classical sand gardens of Japan. These gardens were first created by Buddhist monks as places for quiet reflection. No part of the garden is without meaning; stones and ornaments are arranged in perfect harmony with each other, plants and water features are chosen for their spiritual significance, as well as to inspire the person walking through the garden. The paths are made of gravel or pebbles, and they are raked daily by the monks in traditional formal swirling patterns that convey a deep understanding of and respect for the rhythmic cycles of nature, the ebb and flow of water, the movement of shadows around objects.

Making a miniature sand garden like Randall's is easy. The act of flattening and raking the sand each day, and rearranging the decorative pebbles into new and interesting patterns is calming and meditative.

Zen Garden

> fine coloured sand from craft shops in a silvery grey or pink
> shallow box, e.g. the lid of a shoebox
> small, interestingly shaped rocks or stones
> cake fork

◆ Pour the sand into the box and smooth the surface.

◆ Pick up the stones and allow each one to 'speak' to you. Perhaps it catches the light in a certain way, or that has a more attractive texture than another. Arrange the stones in a way that feels right – in a simple curve or a circle, or a figure-of-eight, or in a close, dense group with one standing alone.

◆ Use the fork to gently rake the sand around the stones; the Zen monks say this balances the male or earth energy of the stones by introducing a female element of water, represented by the sand ripples.

◆ Tend your sand garden for a few minutes each day. Moving the sand and shifting the pieces reminds you that, in nature and in life, everything flows and changes, nothing stays the same.

REMEMBER TO RELAX AND TAKE TIME OUT TO **CREATE** ...

85. CARVE A TOTEM POLE

A shaman is most often described as a medicine man or spirit doctor, and they have existed in nearly all cultures – Native American Indian, Maori, African bushmen and Australian Aboriginal, to name a few. According to shamanic tradition, our lives are intimately connected with plants, animals and spirits, and if we are not acting in harmony with nature, illness and stress will result. So perhaps it isn't surprising that – at this time in modern life, when we are more disconnected from nature than ever before – there has been a resurgence of interest in techniques long practised by shamen, including visualisation, hypnotherapy and meditation.

Traditionally, the shaman was often responsible for giving each person in the tribe or village a symbolic name and assigning a totem that had great power for them. These could be masks, poles, jewellery, belts or breast plates, and they usually depicted animals or events, or natural phenomena which reflected aspects of the individual's personality.

By creating a personal totem pole, you can re-establish your connection with a more natural, spiritual world. Think about what animal inspires you. Is it a horse? A butterfly? An eagle? What colours lift your spirits? Are there symbols that resonate deeply for you, such as a flowerbud, a cross or the sun? The shamanic tradition relies on the idea of individuals creating their own 'story' on their totem as their life develops. Making a totem pole means you are marshalling the powers of all your personal icons so you can face the world in a more grounded, fuller and more fruitful representation of who you are. There is no right or wrong result; your totem is your personal myth and meaning.

TOTEM POLE

a piece of wood measuring 12 cm x 1.5 metres (5 in x 1½ yards)
gloss paint in your favourite colour
glue
tacks
a selection of ribbons, jewels, shells, stars, feathers, etc.

◆ Sand the wood, then paint it. Allow the paint to dry.

◆ Decorate your totem pole by winding on ribbons and gluing or tacking on items that have spiritual or symbolic significance to you, e.g. a spray of feathers for a free spirit, stars and moons for travel, a silk tassel for beauty, a key, a piece of red lace for passion, gold glitter for the sun, a coin for good fortune.

◆ Hang it on your wall where you can see it.

86. MAKE A SCENTED POMANDER

Pomanders can be traced back to the time of the ancient Greeks. In those days they were carried, worn or hung in rooms to counteract the often foul air. Today, they can be hung in the bedroom or wardrobe for sheer pleasure – the scent of a pomander should last at least a year.

Like many simple craft activities, making a traditional pomander is also a deeply soothing activity. The clean, spicy smells of clove, cinnamon and orange are warming and comforting, and the repetitive action of pushing in the clove buds eases your mind while keeping your hands busy. The scents are evocative, and you'll get a deep sense of satisfaction from making something that is pretty, useful and wholesome.

POMANDER

> medium-sized orange
> cloves
> orris root powder (from the chemist)
> ground cinnamon
> narrow ribbon

◆ Use a skewer to prick holes all over the skin of the orange for the cloves. Insert the cloves, as close together as possible, leaving only a cross-shaped space where the ribbon will go around the fruit.

◆ In a bowl, mix together roughly equal quantities of orris root powder and ground cinnamon. Roll the orange thickly in this mixture, making sure it is well covered.

◆ Wrap the orange in a piece of greaseproof paper and leave it for 4 weeks in a dark, dry place. By then, you should have a small, dried-out pomander with a rich citrus smell.

◆ To hang the pomander, tie the ribbon crosswise around it.

87. COLOUR IN

When my children were young they were rarely without crayon or chalk stubs grasped in their sticky little fists, which they would use enthusiastically at every opportunity (the crawl-space underneath the stairs still bears testimony to Ed's fondness for fluorescent Textas and glitter-glue pens).

There is innocent joy and harmony to be found by getting those creative juices flowing, no matter how simple or complex the project you tackle. So, while all forms of painting and drawing are potential outlets for your creativity, just taking a leaf out of the humble colouring-in book will do the trick.

Choose a book with a theme that you enjoy – perhaps flowers or planets, or cartoon characters like Beauty and the Beast. Settle yourself comfortably with a set of coloured pencils, and start to methodically fill in all the shapes, making sure to colour evenly and to not go outside the lines. The key is to bring the full measure of your concentration to your efforts. As you shade evenly and gently, turning the page this way and that, and carefully going over tricky corners, you will find yourself relishing the calm that simple, non-competitive activities bring.

88. DRAW A MANDALA

Mandalas are the highly decorative, symmetrical designs used as a focal point for spiritual contemplation in Buddhism. Most are inspired by nature, and feature the sun or plants, or powerful mystical symbols such as the rose and the cross. Others are based on traditional Tibetan designs. Anyone interested in finding balance, growing in peace and in developing personal awareness through meditation or other spiritual and relaxation exercises will find making a mandala an inspirational and soothing exercise.

MANDALA

> cardboard
> compass
> paints or coloured felt-tip pens

◆ Use the compass to draw a circle about 30 cm (12 in) in diameter on the cardboard. Adjust the compass to draw one or two more smaller concentric circles inside the first. These circles are a symbol of the unfolding of creation from its mystic centre.

◆ Draw outward-travelling spirals, or use a ruler to make straight lines coming out from the central circle. These lines symbolise the sun's rays; they can also represent your own journey to your inner self. Another powerful symbol, which you can use to fill in one or more of the segments, is the oval flower petal – these depict the lotus, which represents beauty growing from mud, just as the spirit rises from confusion to enlightenment and peace.

◆ Colour in your mandala as you please, in soft pastels or bright, striking colours. Use it as a focal point for meditation. If you find it hard to concentrate, keep bringing your attention back to the centre of the mandala, and contemplate the meaning of the different elements which you have drawn: the circles, which suggest the radiating energy in the world which connects us all and the petals, which suggest the renewal of life or perhaps the flowering of your heart. Let them fuse together in your mind, as in the totality of your mandala. Find peace and quiet in this thought.

89. STAMP A POTATO

Did you make potato stamps for printing on paper when you were small? Kids don't have to have all the fun. Nor do you have to be particularly 'artistic' to reap the revitalising benefits of using your hands to make something, to get in touch with your creative side, and have some instant time-out. All you really need is the desire to have a bit of fun.

POTATO-PRINT WRAPPING PAPER

> 3–4 large potatoes, washed
> sharp knife
> poster paints
> butcher's paper or newspaper

◆ Cut the potatoes in half and stand the halves, cut-side down, on a tea-towel for a few minutes to absorb the excess moisture.

◆ With your knife, cut out a pattern on the cut side of each potato. Cross, fish, star, heart, diamond and leaf designs all look great, or even just two simple wavy lines. Scrape out the potato flesh around the design so that you get a raised surface.

◆ Pour about a tablespoonful of paint into a couple of old saucers and dip the potato halves into it. Press lightly onto a sheet of newspaper to get rid of excess paint, then press onto the butcher's paper. Allow to dry thoroughly, then use as inexpensive wrapping paper.

90. TAKE UP WHITTLING

Remember the story of Huckleberry Finn, whittling away at a birchwood twig? Since the beginning of time, men and boys have found it soothing to shave bits off a piece of wood, a little at a time, because – well, just because they can.

As with carving or wood-turning, whittling gives you the sensual pleasure that comes from working with natural materials. The difference is, you don't end up with a piece of furniture or a sculpture; you end up with nothing. There is no point to whittling a piece of wood, which is, of course, the whole point – it gives you time out to think about absolutely nothing.

Whittling wood is a great way to burn off pent-up tension. Take a small, thick stick or a twig and, using a sharp knife, work your way around it, slicing off little bits. Say to yourself: 'That gets rid of you – and you – and you!' The end result? Relaxed hands, relaxed mind, and some wood chips for the garden or compost bin.

91. COME UP WITH A TRADEMARK

You don't have to be a gifted artist to be known for your creativity, or to live a harmonious, inspired life. Everyone can come up with a creative statement, action or motto that reflects their unique personality and nature. Perhaps you already have one trademark activity or habit, or perhaps there are several – what they have in common is that they instantly tell someone else what you stand for and what you believe in.

'Live your beliefs,' wrote the philosopher Henry David Thoreau, 'and you can turn the world around.'

For example, when I think of Suzanne, I think of the fact that she participates in the charity run for breast cancer every year. When I think of Shane, I think of her saying that you should always have a bottle of champagne in your fridge, because there is always something to celebrate. Then there's Carolyn, who made wonderful cross-stitch samplers for all our babies when they were born; Pam, who is famous for her country-style fruitcakes; and Lyn, who always wears a scarf from her extensive collection. And I have worn a gold unicorn – a symbol of truth, courage and love – on a chain around my neck since I was sixteen. A gift from my mother, I wear it to remind me to always act from these intentions.

Being known and remembered for small actions like these say so much more about your beliefs and values. They are the real things about us that make an impact on each other's lives; they are also personal statements in which we can find balance, refocus on what's really important and keep faith with our beliefs.

What one thing can you always be relied upon to do or wear or say? What would you like to be known and remembered for?

'Trust yourself. You know more
than you think you do.'

Dr Benjamin Spock

Grow . . .

Look within and discover your true nature. Self-knowledge is the real source of your moral, emotional and spiritual strength and of your ability to grow as a person. Only when you have made peace with who you are – with your inner self – will you be content with what you have and also with what you do outwardly. Being honest with yourself brings freedom.

Why do some people relish change, movement and growth, while others buckle under pressure and get stuck in a rut? It's all in how we look at things. Those who are resilient seem to rise to a challenge and embrace change instead of fearing it. Self-knowledge and personal growth are not inborn traits, nor are they gifts that are reserved for the old and wise – they are life skills we can all benefit from learning. How you think has a strong effect on your ability to grow and develop, so it's important to adjust your mindset. For example, does criticism depress you, or does it give you an incentive to change your attitude and actions?

Life has many rough edges, and however optimistic or hardworking you are, some things can be difficult to bear or appear impossible to see a way through. Resolving to first understand and hold true to your core values, then to change what you can and accept what you can't, is a good place to start. When changes are based on real self-acceptance and an honest awareness of yourself, your spirit will move freely and be better able to transcend difficulties.

Your intuitive thoughts, feelings and dreams all provide fascinating insight into your habits, behaviour and attitudes. For example, past experiences such as an unfaithful spouse or a miscarriage can colour your reaction to current events and prevent you from dealing with them. Knowing your prejudices and flaws – and forgiving them – can help you recognise habitual responses and face up to things and move forward, instead of backing off and running away.

Acknowledging your anger can help you get rid of it. Understand your emotions and instincts, rather than suppressing them; this can free up vast amounts of energy and passion, and allow you to grow. Life is all the richer when you feel it, rather than fight it, even if that means letting yourself experience regret, anger or shame. Find your truths. Respect yourself as you would like others to respect you, and don't be afraid to try and be a better person.

No matter how many experts you listen to, or how many books you read (including this), the buck stops with you when it comes to taking steps that affect you. Join in the game. Feeling disempowered or stuck only results in frustration and stagnation. Don't make it worse by turning your power over to others. Study your options. Participate, speak up and be involved. Then listen to your inner voice – it's rarely wrong. Ask 'What feels absolutely true and right for me?' Then you – no one else – can decide.

92. FORGIVE YOURSELF

In the Jewish religion, there is a spiritual practice known as kavanna. This can be loosely translated as the desire to live a balanced life: to acknowledge that where there is light, there is also shade, where there is joy, there is also sadness, where there is right, there is wrong.

At Yom Kippur, the annual Jewish festival of atonement, people are asked to remember their sins and misunderstandings from the year just passed. They meditate on them in the spirit of teshuva, which means 'returning to the self'. The idea is not to punish yourself, but to face up to past mistakes and examine them as closely and thoroughly as possible. Then you forgive yourself, and move on.

It is only by acknowledging your errors that you can understand your true self – your motives and your needs – and be free to try once more to press on towards wholeness and harmony, and to grow as a human being. Forgiving yourself means that you release resentment and hostility, two extremely damaging emotions that will compromise your health.

The everyday version of this is to forgive yourself if you don't follow through on your intentions, and to try, try and try again. Albert Schweitzer said, 'A man can only do what a man can do. But if he does that each day he can sleep at night and do it again the next day.' The only way you're going to grow is by going through the experience of falling down and failing – and then getting back up again and having another go.

Self-forgiveness is more than just a one-off act; it is an ongoing process, and one that stops you from holding onto a habit or identity that only festers. Forgiveness may not change the past, but it does open up your future.

93. TAKE ONE STEP AT A TIME

Many centuries ago, the Greek philosopher Ovid wrote, 'Let your hook always be cast because in the smallest pond, where you least expect it, there will be a big fish.' This is a useful image to keep in mind when you are thinking about changing aspects of your life, whether it's your diet, your attitude or your work or family priorities. It's a common mistake to think that, for change to be effective, it has to be something really big and noticeable, and that you have to change everything, all at once. A parallel would be taking up a regular walking practice, and expecting to be fit enough for a half-marathon by the end of the first week. Or signing up for a yoga class and being disappointed if you can't do the lotus position straightaway.

Leo Tolstoy wrote that, 'True life is lived when the tiniest of changes occur.' The pursuit of a calmer, more balanced life is more likely to be made up of many small changes, rather than one or two big ones. It is also the result of a more receptive and observant state of mind, one that is mindful of opportunities for positive change, growth and development. In this way, the most insignificant action – the smallest pond, if you like – can become an opportunity for something significant.

Start with one small change, such as practising a simple visualisation exercise before showering each morning, or lighting a stick of honey incense when you return home in the evening, or swapping coffee for green tea at work. Then add more small changes, and watch them grow into a whole new way of seeing and being every day.

94. BE AN EVERYDAY HERO

When interviewed about his motivation for producing *Million Dollar Baby*, the Academy Award-winning film about a young woman who is determined to become a champion boxer, director Clint Eastwood said he wanted to portray 'the heroism in ordinary people'.

At first glance, these words don't seem to go together. Heroism is more often used to describe behaviour from someone smarter, more famous and generally more important than you, someone who is far away from your everyday life. 'Hero' is the word used for legends and icons such as Mother Teresa, Nelson Mandela, the Dalai Lama, Gandhi, Martin Luther King, all of whom are remembered for their remarkable achievements, leadership qualities, vision and wisdom.

However, we can all be heroes. A teacher arriving at school at 7 a.m. to give a needy child an extra reading lesson is a hero. So are the hundreds of people in a country town protesting peacefully but determinedly against a factory closure.

Heroism is not necessarily about bravery or winning battles. It's about persistence and compassion and the ability to start over again if necessary. Putting your name down to sell a box of badges for the Red Cross fund-raising drive is heroic. So is picking up litter, even if it's not your own, or waiting patiently at a pedestrian crossing for an old person to cross, because they can't move fast enough to keep up with the red signal.

It's not easy being a hero, and it's not realistic to be one 24/7. We all have days when things go wrong, when we lose our temper or fib. Being human means being flawed – we fart, we get hangovers, we get frightened. But it also means having the potential to grow and to change, to behave with integrity rather than selfishness, and to try to make the world a better, safer, happier place.

95. CONCENTRATE ON KEY QUALITIES

Even in the most chaotic and frustrating of times, remember that, deep down, your subconscious knows precisely what you need to do in order to grow, to resolve problems and achieve harmony, and to become calmer.

Many different meditation tools can be used to crystallise your inner thoughts and give you new insight, which propels your progress. Sometimes meditating on a single word is all it takes to trigger that 'Aha!' response, where you sense a breakthrough in understanding that helps shift you forward.

MEDITATION CARDS

> pens or coloured pencils
> ruler
> thin cardboard

◆ Use a pencil and ruler to divide the cardboard into approximately 30 small pieces.

◆ On one side of each piece, write a different word to describe personal qualities and characteristics that you want to develop and focus on in your life. For example: Perseverance, Courage, Humility, Tenderness, Love, Humour, Creativity, Honesty, Tolerance, Generosity, Grace, Acceptance, Flexibility, Optimism.

◆ Put all the cards in a paper bag or envelope and shake it well. Each morning, make it a ritual to close your eyes and take out a card. Read the word, then say it out loud, concentrating hard on what it means to you. What is your first reaction to that word? How does it make you feel? What is something you have done recently that exemplifies it? How can you grow that quality in your life? Aim to do one simple thing that will bring that word to life in the day ahead of you.

96. DAYDREAM

When I was in primary school, I was always getting in trouble for staring out the window, my thoughts filled with mermaids, mythical monsters and fantasies about pirate treasure and fabled explorers. I received good grades, but the faraway look in my eyes infuriated teachers, and my reports are peppered with comments like 'Pamela must concentrate on her work' and 'Could do better if she gave her full attention'.

These words reflect the fashions about thinking and learning at the time I went to school. Students were expected to absorb information by rote, and it was the girl who could recite dates, methods, lists and formulas in perfect order who received the merit awards, not the one who doodled and came up with perplexing questions or unusual ideas. The mind was something to be disciplined and pruned into a formal shape, not something that was allowed to flow and move and grow in directions that weren't planned.

Times change. Psychologists and psychotherapists use free association of words or images to stimulate creativity. Brainstorming is common in both the classroom and the business world as a means of trying to see things from a different perspective, and so being able to pursue new opportunities.

A rich fantasy life can be a source of comfort and inspiration at any age. Daydreaming is a healthy way to release tension, experience playfulness and contemplate free-ranging, abundant possibilities without having to commit to any one in particular.

Dip into a daydream, and see where your mind takes you today.

97. DON'T TRY TO FIX EVERYTHING

Women tend to see themselves as 'fixers'. They feel as though they have to solve problems, change people, get things organised, alter situations, make things better – and they feel they have to do it all within a certain time-frame. However, focusing on a problem – something that has to be fixed, even though it may be beyond your control – is a recipe for stress.

A more productive technique is to train yourself to see that whatever is happening, good or bad, is just information. Learn to paint with a broad brush, to be flexible and see that details will change. Learn from the great US military leader, General Patton, who said he never prepared any battle plan without having at least three alternative back-up plans. If one wasn't working, he'd switch to something else rather than try to force the original idea through.

Instead of responding to problems out of emotion and habit, work through these steps.

◆ **Acknowledge that it's not what you wanted** Simply saying out loud 'Well, I didn't expect that to happen' is enormously powerful because it liberates you from the idea that – somehow – you should have anticipated every possible scenario and outcome, which is, of course, impossible. The only reason a problem is a problem is because you haven't planned for it. It's just something different.

◆ **Give yourself time** Instead of reacting immediately, try to give yourself as much mental processing time as possible. Depending on the situation, this might only be a minute or two, or it could be a couple of days. Rather than feel you have to do something and take action right now, sit back, breathe and wait. See it as an opportunity to gather different information. Ask questions, draw on your experience, look at the issue with different eyes. If you remind yourself to take your time and respond slowly, chances are you'll do and say something much smarter.

◆ **Listen to your inner voice** As you process the information, all sorts of different options will come to mind. Let your intuition guide you towards the one that feels right. If it's a surprising choice, so much the better; the 'right' and logical answer may not always be the best.

98. DECODE YOUR DREAMS

What is a dream? Is it a message from your unconscious mind, which is more insightful than what you see with your conscious mind? Or is it simply the result of your brain neurons firing at random while you sleep?

Vincent van Gogh described dreams as being 'more alive, more richly coloured than waking life'. There are many schools of thought on what a dream is and how it comes about, and there are dozens of books that claim to decode the symbols that appear in dreams. However, only you can describe how a dream makes you feel, and this is how dreaming can be a key to understanding your true inner self – what your deepest desires are, what is lacking in your life, or what is really upsetting you.

A dream diary invites you to explore your own mind. It can also help you to sort out problems and become clearer and calmer in your waking life. Keep a pad of paper and a pen by your bed. As soon as you wake up, write down whatever you can remember dreaming about. It's important not to censor yourself: there is no right or wrong way to do this. For example, you might remember a whole bizarre story in vivid detail, or you might remember a sign, a face, even a smell – or just a strong thought or emotion, such as fear, that may linger for hours.

Keep the dream diary for at least a month. Then look back over your entries and pick out recurring themes or images. Perhaps you always wake with the sense that you are being chased or that you are drowning under water. Or maybe a particular animal or feature keeps turning up, such as a lion or a toilet. Note these patterns and ask yourself what they mean. Why do I feel as though I am being pursued? Who or what am I trying to escape? A toilet means elimination – does this mean there's something in my life I should be trying to get rid of?

99. WAKE UP YOUR SENSES

'It's not the number of senses I have, but what I do with them that is my kingdom,' said Helen Keller. If, for every minute in the day, you are frantically trying to juggle five, ten or fifteen things, then the first casualty will be your sensory awareness. You look without really seeing, eat without really tasting, hear but don't really listen. Days are like blancmange, slipping by unnoticed and unremarkable.

Multi-tasking – which women are so very good at – is a double-edged sword. Being able to tackle several things at once is an important life skill for women who are running a house, a family, holding down a job and possibly caring for aged parents. However, our brains become stressed by this sort of sensory and intellectual overload, which causes anxiety and depression and – ironically – makes us less efficient. This is burnout.

Many personal growth and meditation techniques are based on the idea of focusing attention on one thing at a time. Whether you are eating a peach, drinking a glass of water or hanging out the washing, be fully present and attentive to that activity to really experience it or to learn anything from it, instead of being distracted by something else as well.

Tune in to your senses and give yourself to the moment. Pick up that peach and turn it from side to side, run your thumb over its velvet skin, admire its rosy colour and erotic scent, then bite into its warm, juicy flesh. Drink the water slowly and sensuously: concentrate on the cool temperature, the silky feel as it slips down your throat, the feel of the cold glass on your fingertips. Roll a pebble between your fingertips. Sing in the shower at the top of your voice. Hold your mother's hand, and marvel at the soft, wrinkled skin, the infinitely familiar touch. Sit in the garden with your eyes closed. Wrap yourself in a jewel-coloured mohair rug. Slowly sip homemade soup, and feel it doing you good.

Constantly straining to get ahead, to keep up, to anticipate what you've got to do next – all they do is make you miss the moment you're in. The joy of living a whole and harmonious life is in the palm of your hand – or anywhere you focus your senses – sight, taste, touch, hearing and smell – so that you really notice what is happening to you, right now.

100. FIND YOUR STILL POINT

This technique is ideal if you tend to have a vivid imagination and to be over-analytical, to 'think too much'. It is derived from craniosacral therapy, a branch of osteopathy, which is a system of massage and manipulation that aims to bring the structure of the body back into balance. The philosophy underpinning craniosacral therapy is that, if the spine and neck are correctly aligned, then the body and brain can function properly.

The idea of this exercise is to train your brain to be still, rather than scattered. It works on two levels. First physically, by bringing about a temporary pause – or 'still point' in the fluids that flow through the brain and spinal cord; and then mentally, by replacing the usual jumble of fragrances, sounds, lists and sensations with peaceful, calm images. This technique can help you to live life more consciously, which in turn brings greater control and peace of mind.

Craniosacral therapists use a 'still-point inducer' to prompt this effect, which is usually a small shaped headrest made from wood or plastic. You can substitute this with a plastic dumbbell or place two tennis balls inside a sock and knot the end to hold the balls snugly together. The idea is that the balls will separate slightly when you place your neck on them, but that they will comfortably support your head and allow your airways to be open, not tilted or compressed.

◆ Lie on the floor and notice the spot where the back of your head touches the floor. Briefly lift your head and slide the still-point device under your head, easing the balls slightly apart so your head is 'floating'.

◆ Close your eyes, and let your whole body relax. Take several deep breaths, and recall a special moment when you felt absolutely at peace, e.g. listening to an inspiring piece of music or climbing up to the top of a lighthouse and looking out to sea. Use all your senses to visualise that moment and hold it in your mind, lovingly noticing every detail. Imagine the feelings generated by these thoughts moving out of your head and mind's eye and flowing up and down your spinal cord, filling your whole body. Each time you breathe in, imagine yourself filled with vitality and energy, the way you felt when you first listened to that music or took in that view. As you breathe out, imagine the tension leaving your body.

◆ Rest on the device for 10–15 minutes, continuing to imagine the feelings of peace flowing evenly around your body. Feel your breathing become easier and your muscle tension drop away. If your mind wanders, keep coming back to the image. When you're ready, let the image fade until the next time you need it.

101. CLEAR CLUTTER

If your home is overflowing with clutter, chances are you will also feel as though you can't move or think clearly. The Chinese sage and scholar Lao Tzu wrote, 'He who knows what is enough is free to grow.'

Get rid of stuff you don't need, and get a clear, fresh start so you have space to think and live, and focus on the present.

◆ **Get ready** Write down a phrase that reflects what you want, such as 'I want to move forward and be more in control of my life'. Keep saying it. Pick a time when you have a block of three or four hours. Choose an area or a cupboard that has been annoying you the most. Have at least four strong garbage bags or big cardboard boxes handy. Label them 'Rubbish', 'Recycle', 'Give Away' and 'Belongs Elsewhere'.

◆ **Start sorting** The golden rule is to put like with like, whether it's CDs, socks or saucepans. Start with the category that will clear the biggest space – it'll motivate you. Finish one cupboard, corner or room before moving on to the next. Be firm: decide what to keep and what to put in your 'Give Away' and 'Belongs Elsewhere' boxes. Ditch everything that's not necessary or beautiful. Acknowledge that you will have to face up to emotional baggage. For example, different possessions may make you feel sad, sentimental or just plain furious. That's fine. Let the feelings bubble up and release.

◆ **Put it away** Have a designated place to put things, and ensure your system matches the way you actually move in and use that particular space. Most importantly, stop it from happening all over again. Stuff will keep coming in – you just have to keep sending it back out. Bring in only what you really want, love or need.

102. LEARN TO READ AGAIN

During any average week, you might read between 5000 and 10 000 words. Add up all the newspapers, real estate blurbs, television programs, office notices, supermarket special brochures, school newsletters and notes and you'll see it's not hard to get to that figure.

However, very few of those words will inspire your spirit or stimulate your mind. And, if you're studying for an exam, or if your work means you spend a lot of time reading reports or analysing documents, the figure can climb even higher, but your brain will subconsciously associate reading of any sort with work and stress.

Watch the expression on the face of a child who is completely absorbed in a book. The Jewish philosopher Martin Buber wrote, 'Youth is the time of total openness. With totally open senses, a child absorbs the world's variegated abundance. He has not yet sworn allegiance to any one truth.' Think back to those lazy moments in your childhood where you stretched out on your stomach on the grass to read myths and legends, or when you curled up in a favourite chair to escape through a magic door with goblins, griffins and princesses. For many children, learning to read opens the door to a world of infinite possibilities and ideas.

Learn to read – again – and rediscover the joy of getting completely absorbed in a vivid, imaginative story. Choose a book that is the opposite of what you would usually pick. Instead of a murder mystery, try a romance or something by a new science fiction writer. And it's never too late to read children's novels, either – classics like *The Snow Goose*, *Charlotte's Web*, *I Capture the Castle* and *Little Women* aren't just for children; they appeal to people of all ages because they are wonderfully entertaining and uplifting.

103. BUST YOUR RUT

'The one thing you think you can't change? That's the thing you must change,' said Eleanor Roosevelt. A routine is only one step away from a rut. When you do the same things day after relentless day, you become bored. You feel stiff, dried-up and stuck, less alive.

Every day presents hundreds of possibilities for doing things differently and for growing as a person – listening to new music, taking a different route to work, trying something unusual for dinner. When you make even one small change to a routine, you instantly feel more connected, more juiced. However, we humans are notoriously reluctant to make even little changes like these. A habit or behaviour can be causing us actual physical pain or emotional damage, but we still manage to justify it and to grimly hang on to it. The habits then define our limitations, because the world is only as big as what you allow yourself to know.

Consider activities in your day where habit is most evident: the way you store food in the cupboard, or a system of reporting that you follow at work, for example. Now, do that activity with fresh eyes, as though you had never done it before. Think about how you use the cupboard, and arrange the food differently. Think about who will be reading the report you're preparing, and whether there's a smarter, more appropriate way of setting it out.

Habits can slowly squeeze the life out of relationships, too, locking you into a loop of actions or thoughts. For example, perhaps there is a work acquaintance you regard as rude or untrustworthy. Your opinion hardens into a habitual pattern of behaviour, as you speak to them in a particular way, or avoid them altogether. You may think that this is a protective mechanism, but it's actually stopping you from growing, because it prevents you from looking at each moment, event and person with fresh eyes. You feel no need to look within yourself for a different perspective, or perhaps for more patience, tolerance or courage.

You don't need to sign up for an adrenalin-pumped adventure to break out of a rut. Just look at things differently, and become aware of the consequences of small daily actions that may be limiting – this will allow you growth and new perspective. Marcel Proust said, 'The voyage to self-discovery is not through new landscapes, but through new eyes.'

104. WRITE YOUR OWN LIFE

If you're feeling stressed and overwhelmed, it's easy to feel inadequate as well, to get bogged down in the dull minutiae of daily life rather than to see the 'big picture'.

Imagine that you've written a book, and the publisher has asked you to prepare a brief biographical note for the cover flap. What would you include? It wouldn't be the fact that you have to remember to collect the dry-cleaning today. Nor would it be the appointment with your child's English teacher tomorrow, or even the family get-together on the weekend. If you had to describe yourself in just a few sentences, chances are you'd focus on positive things that have happened to you – your achievements, your personality and perhaps your hopes and dreams.

Pretending to write a biography for the cover flap of your book is a quick and easy way to take stock of where you're at in your life. Take one minute (and it must be only one) to describe yourself. Do it straight away: You must not stop to take a break or think of words different from the first ones that pop into your head, because it's those first phrases that are the most insightful.

While it's a fun thing to do, like many of the ideas in this book, it's deceptively powerful, and helps you to acknowledge your strengths. The writing task also forces you to be concise; when you only have a limited time to write, what's really important to you becomes very clear.

One tip is to try to move past the obvious. The interesting thing about this exercise is how it throws up the characteristics and dreams that tend to get buried beneath the usual ways that you describe and define yourself – what you look like, where you live, what you do. For example, instead of 'I am a 40-year-old mum who works part-time at the local school', write 'I am tenacious, honourable and hardworking. I am a loyal friend, and I will fight to the death for my children. I love my home, but I'd still like to sail away. I would love to live close to the ocean.'

Put your description somewhere you can read it when you have those days where you think you're only capable of stuffing the same envelope over and over again. Stick it on the fridge door, or write it in your diary. Read it out loud to remind yourself of who you really are.

105. EMBRACE CHANGE

If you regard a change as a threat, as something you're not capable of managing, or even as a major headache in your life, you will become frightened of it. Dolly Parton said, 'The way I see it, if you want to have the rainbow, you gotta take the rain as well.' So, if you accept that change is a natural part of your life, and that it's an opportunity for you to learn or to grow, then you're more likely to face up to the fear and see the challenges that come your way as exciting possibilities, rather than as dramas.

An easy way to make sense of your fears is to remember that you don't have control over everything and everyone in your life – the rain and the rainbow, if you like – but you do have control over the way you react to them. For example, you don't have control over your boss's mood swings, but you do have control over whether you allow yourself to be upset by them. Only rarely can a person or a situation actually force you to feel a certain way. It is the meaning that you place on that person or situation – how you think about it, not what they think about you – that results in what you feel. In short, your emotions are the direct result of how you perceive the world. Once you try this highly effective way of facing up to your fears, a more flexible way of thinking will result, and commonsense and truth are usually revealed.

Next time you feel frightened, follow these steps.

◆ **Name the feeling** Were you really frightened? Or were you sad, tired or surprised?

◆ **Note the way you reacted physically** Did you feel sick in the stomach? Or develop a headache, or cry?

◆ **Identify the trigger** A bank statement, an unexpected deadline?

If you take these cognitive steps you won't see whatever happened as a frightening catastrophe, but as something that you can embrace and handle. Then, instead of hiding behind negative self-talk such as 'This is going to be a disaster, nothing ever works out for me', step right up to the fear in your mind's eye and say to yourself, 'This is what has happened. What can I learn from it.' Straight away, the problem becomes smaller and you will feel more centred, less overwhelmed.

106. BE PROUD OF YOUR STRENGTHS

For decades, fashion and beauty magazines have made millions of dollars out of women's tendency to focus on the perceived shortcomings in their appearances, rather than on their unique talents. It is a habit that easily spills over into other aspects of life, fuelling insecurity and arresting your development as a person. It is a negative exercise and largely a futile one.

Abraham Lincoln wrote, 'People are about as happy as they make up their minds to be.' So instead of dwelling on overcoming what you perceive as weaknesses that make you unhappy and discontented (for example, 'I'm so disorganised' or 'I have a dreadful temper'), spend more energy thinking about your strengths ('I'm a good listener', 'I have a gift for languages'). Thinking of your weak points does nothing for you – worse, it just feeds your lack of self-worth and gives you excuses for not taking up challenges and seeking solutions.

If you don't know what your strengths are, pay attention to what you're doing when you have a smile on your face, or when time flies by because you are so absorbed in a task. Make a list of these activities and skills, then break them down into smaller details. For example, don't just write 'I enjoy being a teacher'. Instead, write 'I like the energy of being around young children', 'I know how to comfort someone who's feeling confused' and 'I am good at explaining things'. Describe your strengths in detail.

Seeing yourself in terms of your gifts and abilities gives you a sense of purpose. People who focus on their strengths, rather than their weaknesses, have a reason to get up each day and they are always moving forward.

107. GET GOOD AND MAD

Men are more likely to cite feeling out of control in a situation as a reason for getting angry, while women say that having too many demands on their time is what causes them to see red. I have always had a hard time even acknowledging that I'm really cross about something, let alone expressing it, having come from a long line of women who have been instructed since babyhood to maintain a pleasant façade despite boiling with rage on the inside.

Getting angry every so often is, in fact, a very healthy thing to do, while keeping it all pent up inside is not. Understanding how you deal with anger – or how you don't deal with it – can help you grow out of destructive patterns in your personal and professional relationships and move forward. These ideas will help you vent your vexation more constructively.

◆ **Take a break** Anger arouses us, lowering inhibitions and leading us to blurt out things we later regret. In the heat of the moment, do something to clear your head: go for a walk, slowly sip some iced water or lock yourself in the bathroom for 5 minutes of deep breathing.

◆ **Get physical** Vigorous exercise is a great way to discharge aggressive feelings, whether it's taking a boxercise class or belting a few golfballs around at the driving range. Even kicking a cardboard box around the room or thumping a pillow or cushion helps release negative emotions.

◆ **Make a noise** Sit and hum. Concentrate on feeling the sound resonate through your body. Or tune in to some upbeat music and sing along – really belt it out. Long, noisy sighs, outraged screams, and deep grunts and groans all help release emotional tension. Get out in the kitchen and rattle those pots and pans. Crash some saucepan lids together as long and hard and noisily as you like. Making noise releases pent-up frustration, fury and disappointment, and helps your body relax by creating feel-good endorphins in your brain.

◆ **Appoint an anger buddy** Find someone trustworthy you can call or email to blow off steam. Make a pact that you can each share your most intimate thoughts without feeling judged or having the other person 'fix' or attempt to explain your feelings away.

108. KNOW THAT YOU ARE LOVED

The most important things in your life aren't things – they're people. Your family and friends may be close by or live with you, or they may be far away, or not even living anymore. However, the fact that they have loved you and supported you and that you have shared positive experiences with them is part of who you are.

Oscar Wilde wrote, 'The aspects of people that are most important to us are hidden because of their familiarity'. Because they are familiar, we tend to discount them. Keep your loved ones close at hand. The most obvious way to do this is with a collection of photographs of family members, friends, teachers or other significant mentors. Other sentimental items may remind you of a special time you spent together, or a quality about that person that is important to you, that gives you strength or in some way steadies you each time you use it or notice it.

For example, I keep a very old, rose-patterned cup that belonged to my grandmother, and I always use it for cracking eggs when baking, just as she did. Every time I pick it up, I immediately see her at her kitchen table cutting out cookie dough, the sunlight coming in the window behind her. My dad's war medals and my mother's thimble are always in a box on my desk for the same reason; it helps me to sense their presence on even the most despairing of days. I also keep my dad's old watch there, and I will often run my thumb over the wristband and breathe in the long-ago scent of leather and Old Spice.

Simple, everyday things can remind us of special people, and these memories have the power to lift us in times of stress. Keep mementoes close by that will bring comfort and remind you that you are loved.

109. WRITE A DIARY

'Face your mind's demons, and they become nothing but shadows', says a traditional Samurai proverb. When you are feeling confused or are face-to-face with a crisis, writing about your feelings can help to neutralise the negative emotions, and provide an inspirational record of your growth and development through good and bad experiences.

Writing about your thoughts and ideas also has a significant effect on your physical health. Studies of cancer patients have demonstrated that the ones who explored their feelings in a journal had significantly fewer medical appointments; they also reported enhanced vigour and decreased fear. Writing about their experience took the raw edge off their feelings, so the trauma carried less negative power.

Most of us can benefit and grow from a little self-examination. Writing down your thoughts and feelings regularly – however briefly – is a way of strengthening your sense of self and sorting out what was worthwhile and nourishing in your day from what people or events brought you down. Committing thoughts to paper (or to a computer file) and working through any problems you identify makes the problems more real – which also makes them more manageable, rather than elusive 'demons'.

It does not matter if you don't solve a problem right away. Simply getting it out of your head is progress and will help you to feel calmer. Your journal is a safe and forgiving place, one where you can scream, rant and complain, and gather the strength you need in order to go back out into the world again tomorrow.

Try setting an egg-timer or stopwatch and just writing whatever pops into your head during that time. The most important aspect of writing in a diary or journal is to release pent-up tension and to acknowledge your feelings. However, you'll also find it interesting and surprising to go back over your notes in months and years to come and see how you are changing.

To be a successful diarist, try to be as honest as you can. Look for patterns and recurrent themes in your writing. A diary is a powerful tool for personal growth. You can look back and note a previous reaction to a situation so that when you're faced with a similar scenario, you can consciously react in a different, more productive way.

110. CHANGE YOUR MOOD WITH MUSIC

People respond to music in a highly individual way: what you find soothing and relaxing, someone else may find intensely irritating. Music is the quickest way to the heart, and a song – or even a single opening note – can propel you instantly to a particular place and time, and bring to life the emotional experiences you had there.

Music with a slow, rhythmic tempo is usually best for deep relaxation. Simple, pure sounds, such as the flute and harp, can have an uplifting effect on the spirit. Much of the ambient music designed to assist meditation and relaxation incorporates instruments that provide long, sustained, soothing notes such as temple bells or chimes, along with sounds from nature such as bird calls and waves. The comfortable, intimate sound of jazz can also help you chill out, as can floating, gentle piano solos that touch the heart.

Here are some chill-out favourites from my music library.

- Chuck Mangione, *Feel So Good*

- Dan Fogelberg and Tim Weisberg, *Twin Sons of Different Mothers*

- George Benson, *Breezin'*

- Art Garfunkel, *Angel Clare*

- Stan Getz and Joao Gilberto, *Getz/Gilberto*

- Norah Jones, *Come Away with Me*

- Diana Krall, *Live in Paris*

- Andrea Bocelli, *Romanza*

- Johann Pachelbel, *Canon in D*

- Ravel, *Pavane for a Dead Princess*

- The complete Nocturnes by Chopin, and Mozart's Piano Concertos, especially numbers 23 and 24

Relax, sit back, and let the music open your mind and take you wherever you want to go.

111. COLOUR YOUR WORLD

Colours have profound effects on your emotions, stress levels, blood pressure and how you see the world. They can stimulate and energise you, making you move and think faster, and they can help you to slow down, feel more relaxed and increase your ability to concentrate.

Think about the colours that you wear and surround yourself with. Even a tiny change can make all the difference to your mood.

◆ **Red** Feeling tired or need a creative boost? Wear red. Stimulating and strengthening, it is said to stimulate appetite and restore physical and mental vitality. It's also the colour we associate with passion and sexual energy.

◆ **Orange** Similar to red in that it is stimulating, orange will create a sense of warmth, comfort and positive energy.

◆ **Yellow** If clarity of thought is what you need, wearing yellow will help you to be rational yet emotionally integrated. Inspirational and uplifting, it lightens mood and helps you concentrate and communicate.

◆ **Green** If you are unsettled, wear green to regain inner balance and equilibrium. It is the colour of nature and so has soothing and healing qualities. It is symbolic of growth and fertility.

◆ **Blue** Do you have a speech or an important presentation to make? Wear blue, the colour of authentic communication. Gentle, calming and relaxing, blue creates a sense of free and clear vision, which is why it has been traditionally used in religious art as a symbol of truth and higher wisdom.

◆ **Purple** Soothing and settling to the nerves, purple has also been much used in religious and spiritual practice because it is a colour thought to enhance psychic abilities, including clairvoyance.

◆ **White** Creates a feeling of simplicity, light and peace.

112. DON'T TAKE LIFE TOO SERIOUSLY

Mark Twain said, 'Time spent laughing is time spent with the gods'.

Laughter is the quickest way to restore a sense of balance and harmony, and to establish an authentic connection with others. A smile or a laugh defuses a tense situation, relaxes you, lifts your spirits, restores your sense of context and helps you to accept mistakes.

Laughter really is 'the best medicine' for your physical health; studies show that a depressed mood triggers hormones that suppress immune activity, while the more you laugh, the more antibodies you produce. A good laugh also releases endorphins, the body's 'feel good' hormones.

Look for the upside in everything. Learn to laugh at yourself. Use humour and play as daily coping strategies to keep you calm and focused, and to release tension. Discover what makes you smile and what makes you laugh, and keep a few triggers handy. These could be a book of cartoons, a comic video, funny cards or some images you can call to mind. My favourite is watching game shows with the kids. We yell out whatever answers come to mind, and laugh when we're right, and laugh when we're wrong.

The bonus is that smiling and laughter are infectious, so by lightening your own day you can also lighten the day of those around you. Laughter is a warm wind and soft wine for your soul.

113. SEE WORK AS A JOURNEY

Sometimes being stressed at work isn't the problem. It's the way you approach your work that defines how much – or if – you enjoy it, and how well you cope with different situations. According to one study from the American Institute of Stress, no one job is necessarily more stressful than others; it's how a person perceives their job that counts.

It's easy to get fixated on surface appearances over work – to worry about a missed deadline or being passed over for a particular position – and to see your progress in a very limited way as a result. Our culture also encourages us to see work in a linear fashion, as a 'career path' that moves from point A to B, via a neat pattern of stepping stones labelled with different job titles and accomplishments.

Rather than seeing work as an artificial template that you have to cut your life to fit, it helps to regard work as a natural, organic river weaving through your life. By acknowledging the contradictions, the shades of grey, the ups and downs, the cycles and the flow from past to future, you gain a more balanced and relaxed view of your work.

This also releases you from the thousands of negative comments that you say to yourself each and every day. This self-talk is often unconscious and can heavily influence how you see yourself and your accomplishments. Start to monitor your self-talk by saying positive things about yourself – 'You are a hardworking, honest and loyal employee' or 'You can manage this project, one step at a time' and see how your mind and body react. That missed deadline then becomes an opportunity to redo an assignment in a new and better way, while the lost promotion becomes a chance to change direction and retrain for a completely different profession.

Look on obstacles as opportunities and setbacks as fresh starts that will help you to see the deeper meaning behind everything you do. Author Joseph Campbell writes that 'what we are really seeking is an experience of being alive at all times, so that all our life experiences resonate with our innermost being and reality'. Learning to see your work in shades of grey rather than in black-or-white absolutes means all your waking hours are an opportunity to feel fully alive, not just the ones when you're not at work.

Bring your whole mind to whatever you are doing. Tackle tasks with all your energy, throw yourself into them. As with any relationship where you invest positive energy and willpower, you will receive a greater return in terms of satisfaction and fulfilment. When you use all your effort and push through old habits and boundaries, the satisfaction you gain is its own reward.

Train yourself to become absorbed in the activity itself, not the outcome. People who say they love their work invariably find that when they are so absorbed in what they are doing, they lose all sense of time and place. Athletes also feel this when they're 'in the zone' and artists often experience it during the creative process.

Experiencing this flow at work is a skill that you can develop, and it is the key to satisfaction, no matter what the job. Being able to find happiness in a task despite emotional trauma or physical setbacks is your right, and it strengthens your ability to concentrate and be consciously creative enough to get lost in the joy of being alive. As with everything else in life, the journey of work matters more than the destination. Enjoy your trip.

114. CREATE A ZEN OFFICE

Change the way you think about what you do. These mind tricks help create harmony and order so you can handle crises better and tackle the day's activities serenely.

◆ **Affirm yourself** You are more likely to achieve your goals if you think positively rather than negatively. Affirmations work on the idea that the verbal or mental repetition of a positive phrase is stated as though it were fact – visualise your situation as you would like it to be. The idea is, you create your own reality by how you think. For example, 'I can cope with challenges', 'I will take one step at a time' or even 'I will breathe deeply and calmly. (Or – one for really bad days – 'It could be worse: I could be related to these people.')

◆ **Step sideways** Pablo Picasso declared that 'the chief enemy of creativity is boredom'. If you feel bored, mentally step sideways and look at approaching your work from a different angle. Sometimes 'creativity' is just a case of reworking what is already there and doing it differently. Did you know, for example, that although shoes have been around for centuries, the idea of having a left- and right-shaped sole was only developed 100 years ago?

◆ **Keep a CD in your computer** Pop on earphones and chill out, even if it's just for a moment. Music has a profound and immediate effect, helping to slow your heart rate, lower your blood pressure, and inspire, energise or relax you.

◆ **Take a break from email** Instead of emailing your colleague on the floor above, go and talk to him or her face-to-face, or use the phone. Unlike email, talking allows you to discuss unrelated subjects, and to notice facial expressions and body language, all of which help you to connect with others in a more balanced, realistic way.

◆ **Inhale peace** Gandhi wrote that 'peace and balance result when what you think, do and say are all in harmony'. This mini-meditation can be done any time at work. Sit quietly, focus on your breath and slowly inhale, visualising your lungs filling with oxygen. Exhale and relax your shoulders. Repeat. Next, slowly say to yourself 'I am' as you inhale and 'at peace' as you exhale. Feel a sense of peace settle around you as what you are saying, doing and thinking become one.

◆ **Think white thoughts** Train your mind to stop swinging to habitual reactions and 'red thoughts' that inflame your emotions and drive up your blood pressure, such as 'I'll get him for this' or 'She's such an idiot for doing that'. Instead, practise 'white' alternatives, such as 'I will look for another way to make him see things as I do' or 'I won't try talking to her now, I'll wait until I'm calmer'.

◆ **See it happen** 'Whether you think you will succeed or not, you're right', said Henry Ford. Athletes are trained to envisage their goals, to not only think that they can achieve their aim, but to actually *see* themselves succeeding by touching the pool wall first, or scoring a goal before they've kicked the ball. Before heading into a tough meeting, visualise yourself achieving the successful outcome you want, and hold the feeling in your mind as you enter the room.

◆ **Find a touchstone** It could be a water cooler, a picture, a pot plant – something tangible that you walk by regularly during your day. Imagine that, every time you see it, it is telling you to take a deep breath, to take a two-minute break, or even to smile more at your colleagues. Make a point of putting your hand on it every time you pass, and keep it there for the length of a breath. Psychologists call this technique 'anchoring', because it helps you slow down and stay calm, clear and focused.

115. RESPECT YOURSELF

'Do unto others as you would be done by – or be done by as you did', wrote Charles Kingsley in *The Water Babies*.

In fact, the first part of living by this golden rule is to treat yourself well. If you don't, you won't know how to treat others well, either.

You can't make others happy or calm or contented if you treat yourself in a negative, critical way. The things you tell yourself have an impact on your mood and on your body. Not only do negative thoughts trigger the release of stress hormones in your body, they also turn up the volume on the 'movie' of harsh self-criticism that is running endlessly in your head, determining your reaction to situations. For example, you might get angry with your child for a good reason, but this turns up the volume on the 'movie' that is constantly saying 'I'm a terrible mother. Those kids would be better off without me'.

If you're sabotaging your chances for contentment and inner peace with this kind of disrespectful talk, resolve to speak to yourself more kindly, as you would to a good friend. Pay close attention to your thoughts, and when you find yourself having a negative thought, replace it with a positive one. Still thinking of it in 'movie' terms, simply start typing in a new, kinder subtitle. 'I'm a normal mother. It's OK to get exasperated every so often – it doesn't mean I don't love my kids.'

If you find this new thinking difficult, try an audiotape or CD of positive affirmations to rewind your mind. You may find that listening to positive, nurturing statements once or twice a day for several weeks is all it takes to train you to speak more respectfully to yourself. Write down the statements that resonate strongly with you. 'I will treat myself calmly and patiently', 'I will travel through my day peacefully' and 'If I feel overwhelmed, I will take a break' are simple and effective ones to try.

116. MEET YOUR INNER AMAZON

My mother comes from a long line of pioneering stock: stubborn, red-headed, stout-booted women who could crack a snake's head in one hand while delivering a baby with the other. Mum has always told me that being strong doesn't mean being heavy-handed or a bully – it just means being confident in yourself, in your capabilities and your rights.

This belief is echoed in the writings of martial arts master and philosopher Sun Tzu: 'If you know yourself, you need not fear the result of a hundred battles'. Finding that steely inner core, that quiet point at your centre that says 'I will bend, but not break' is a critical step towards growth and maturity as a human being. For one thing, it means you know, deep down, that you are capable of defending yourself, and of not buckling under pressure. It also means that you know that you can get a job done and follow through to the end. There is no need to panic or feel unsure.

If you're feeling insecure or unsure about your abilities, tune in to your inner Amazon with this tai chi sequence, the Warrior. It is said to focus your thoughts and channel your mental and physical energies.

◆ Stand up and take a step to your left so your legs are slightly more than hip-width apart.

◆ Bend your knees, lowering your hips, keeping your knees and toes aligned, so you look as though you are astride a horse.

◆ Cross your wrists in front of your chest, with your right arm on the outside, palms facing out.

◆ Maintaining the stance, extend your left arm in line with the shoulder, forefinger pointing up, thumb stretched back and other fingers bent. At the same time, make a fist with the right hand and lift the right arm to shoulder height as if drawing a bow; look at your left hand. Imagine the problem is being 'shot' away from your left hand as you release the 'bow'. Feel the strength in your legs, feel your lungs expanding and filling with air.

◆ Return to the starting position and repeat, alternating sides.

117. NOTICE THE LITTLE THINGS

Aesop wrote, 'Nothing small is ever insignificant – even the tiniest act of gratitude or pure thought is never wasted'.

Small kindnesses, treats and quiet pleasures – it's the little things in life that matter. They are your key to harmony, growth and happiness, not the big, splashy, obvious events.

Small joys and comforts are what expand your mind, warm your heart and feed your spirit. They take you to a healthier, simpler head space, one beyond limitations imposed by belief patterns, habits, money, lifestyle choices, other people's expectations, shoulds and shouldn'ts, and past hurts or embarrassments.

Get into the habit of finding at least three small joys or comforts that you appreciate each day. Perhaps you loved the luxurious feeling of the cherry-red cashmere scarf that you snuggled around your throat this morning. Maybe your partner brushed your hair or gave you an extra-special cuddle. Or you had a nap in the sun at lunch-time, or bought a bunch of bright yellow daisies. Perhaps, when you picked up bread and milk, a stranger opened the shop door for you because your hands were full. Or you saw a beautiful watercolour in the window of an art gallery on the way home, or were able to have fresh figs and yoghurt for breakfast.

You can jot down your three things in your diary, or put them on a post-it note and stick it on the fridge door as a reminder of all that you have in your life that you can be grateful for. Or you might want to make it into a daily ritual where you say them aloud or in your mind just before sleeping. On a bad day, you might only come up with one or two things that happened, but at least try to think about them in as much detail as possible. For example, rather than just saying or writing 'I'm grateful for the fresh figs and yoghurt today', really relish the thought of them. How did they taste and feel on your tongue? Think about the gorgeous purple and green colour of the figs and how they contrasted with the creamy yoghurt. Think about how they nourished you and did you good.

You'll find that happiness is not just in these little things themselves; it's in all the details surrounding them that you would normally skim over. You'll find an infinite source of pleasure and contentment if you train yourself to really notice the positive, uplifting little things that are all around you, every day of your life.

118. WRITE A 'BEFORE I DIE' LIST

Mark Twain wrote, 'Twenty years from now you will be more disappointed by the things you didn't do than by the ones you did. So throw off the bowlines, sail away from the safe harbour. Catch the trade winds in your sails. Explore. Dream. Discover.' To see if your life is 'out there somewhere' or present in the here and now, ask yourself, 'If I died tomorrow, what would I regret not having done? What have I put on hold? What am I waiting for?'

Setting goals – rather than just tentatively wishing and hoping – invites new possibilities. It helps us to grow as human beings: when you are living to your heart's desire, it's easy to be glad for people who are doing the same thing. If you're not, you're more likely to feel jealous and bitter.

Be bold. Write down every dream, every idea you've ever thought you'd like to try. They can be as large or as small as you wish, but you must write them all. Timidity limits you, so even if a goal seems overwhelming ('Take a cruise through the fjords of Norway'), writing it down means you have at least taken that first baby step towards achieving it.

Take your time and don't censor yourself. If learning scuba-diving comes to mind, write it down before your logical mind leaps in and says 'Don't be silly, of course you can't'. Same goes for 'Go away with Dad for a weekend for his seventieth birthday', 'Look up Mrs Arshard from third class', 'Buy a pianola', 'See the Whitsundays', 'Paint dining room cherry-red', 'Learn glass-making', 'Go to Japan' and 'Take the kids to Disneyland'.

Life coaches the world over agree that we are a mission-specific species. When we don't have a goal or plan in front of us, we become disorganised and depressed. Set short- and long-term goals to provide focus and clarity. At the heart of goal-setting – whether it's a daily 'to do' list or one for your whole life – is having a clear purpose in life, and taking joy in taking charge.

Break down major goals into shorter, feasible steps. Every week or month, review what you've written. Cross off things you've achieved, and set new goals. Because these are personal dreams and fancies – as opposed to more serious goals like having financial security – you can cross things off that no longer appeal, or which have been superseded. Just make sure that if you delete 'Get a tattoo' it's because you're not interested any more, not because you're worried about what your mother will think.

119. NAME YOUR FEARS

Finish this sentence: 'The thing I worry most about happening is …' Write down your answer and look at it.

Now, what hard evidence do you have that this thing you're worried about will actually happen? For example, if your answer was 'Losing my job and not being able to pay the mortgage', has your boss given you cause to believe that your work is not up to standard? Assuming this is so (it probably isn't), would it be possible to refinance your home? By questioning your emotive response, you are better able to face realistic fears and to look at unfounded ones in a more rational way.

The next step is to reprogram yourself to react in a different way. Remember the word-association games you played in primary school, where the teacher would say a word and you had to write down the first word that came to your mind? You can use the same technique to gently probe an answer to a problem where your feelings are paralysed by fear.

- Close your eyes and think once again of the fear you have already named.

- Open your eyes and write on a piece of paper, 'But deep in my heart I believe that …' Then write your answer.

- Repeat the exercise at least three times – first closing your eyes and concentrating, then writing the word or phrase that is deep in your heart. Depending on how entrenched your fear is, you may struggle through a few stages, and end up with something like this: 'The thing I worry about most is losing my job. But deep in my heart, I know that I would cope if it happened. Deep in my heart, I know that my real fear is that I don't want to be rejected as being too old. But deep in my heart, I know that even if this did happen, it would be their loss, because I am very capable. And deep in my heart I know that if I did have to find another job I would.'

This exercise is a powerful way to focus on your real fears and prejudices; you will invariably find that the first fear you name is actually a smokescreen. It is a relief to see the underlying one written down. Shakespeare said, 'Know thy enemy'. When your real fear is finally outed, you know what it is you have to purge yourself of.

120. GET A NEW PERSPECTIVE ON MONEY

Facing up to your financial obligations and shifting your perceptions about money to a more balanced perspective will help you cope better with everyday financial ups and downs. Here's how.

◆ **Work out your real worth** List all your non-financial achievements and experiences, such as having children, studying and travelling. Your assets should include all the things you've invested time and energy in, and all the lessons you've learned about life that you can pass on to others. Acknowledge that you are rich in ways you don't realise.

◆ **Question your beliefs** Take a pen and list the first three thoughts that come into your head when you think of money. Now ask, 'Are these facts or opinions?' Chances are they are opinions you have picked up from friends and family. Even seemingly worthy ones such as 'If you work hard, you'll get ahead financially' are not necessarily true.

◆ **Give it away** When you use a portion of what you have – no matter how small – to help others and so to change the world around you, that is when you experience true wealth. Whether you're donating $2 to a breast cancer fund-raiser, or investing in an environmentally sustainable company, ensure your money is aligned with what you believe in.

◆ **You have enough** See consumerism for what it is – a pointless, never-ending exercise in greed. Keep spending simple and you instantly remove a great source of stress. Be one of the 'wanna have it, gotta have it' group and you'll set yourself up for a lifetime of discontent. Acknowledge who you are, what you like, but also what you can afford. Shift your focus from things you don't have to things that you do. Wealth is not about having what you want – it's wanting what you already have.

◆ **Free yourself from debt** Debt is a bondage that restricts you from growing, because it sours your spirit and limits your choices. Cut up the credit cards and set in place a program for paying off the balances; a financial counsellor can help.

121. BELIEVE IN SOMETHING

Frank Lloyd Wright said it perfectly: 'I believe in God – I just call it Nature'.

You can believe in something religious, but you don't have to. For example, you might believe in preserving rainforests or pygmy flying possums or in the importance of family. The crucial thing is that you believe in something outside of yourself, have something that sustains your spirit.

We live in a time of cynicism and mistrust, and we are increasingly isolated from other people. Now, more than ever, it's important to connect with others who believe in the same things. The word 'religion' actually comes from Latin words meaning 'to join' and 'to become one', which explains why churches, synagogues, temples, mosques – indeed, all faiths in one form or another – have traditionally preached a message of joining with a universal power, of becoming one with a great spirit.

You may choose not to believe in all the attendant rituals and festivals, but even the act of looking at different belief systems provides many opportunities for personal growth and for making sense of your own thoughts and life. Do some research in your local library or use the Web to study different religions.

Practise praying. You don't have to get down on your knees if you don't want to, and sanctuary and serenity are always on offer at any sacred space near you. Praying can be done in many ways, such as chanting, singing, walking or sitting quietly. It gives you time out to travel within, focus on what's important in your life, regroup, relax, and be better prepared to go forward and put your heart's desire into action.

122. GO ON A PILGRIMAGE

All the great cultures of the world have traditions of travelling to holy shrines or other places thought to encourage spiritual growth and meditation, or even to facilitate miraculous change. This does not mean that you have to start packing for Mecca or Lourdes. However, you can turn even the shortest time-out into something more restorative and healing if you choose a destination that will replenish your spirit in some way, rather than just somewhere that will entertain and distract you.

It is important to differentiate a pilgrimage from a regular holiday. Perhaps you are due for six months' worth of long-service leave from work, or you are just coming up to another weekend. Irrespective of how much time you have, resolve to make the break more enriching and use the time to grow and develop as a person. Time away from job stress and routine will help you stay mentally and physically alert, too.

During your time off, slow down and work through thoughts and ideas and memories. For example, it could be an overnight silent retreat: go to a bed-and-breakfast, and plan to rest, sleep and walk, quite alone, for twenty-four hours. Take books, perhaps, but promise yourself that you will spend the time in quiet contemplation, and not turn on the TV or dash around taking photographs. Or it could be an afternoon visit to an aged friend or relative, or a tour of a nearby temple or ancient rock paintings, or of some other place with a strong spiritual essence.

At the other end of the scale, your pilgrimage could be a deeply personal, even sentimental, trip of a lifetime. For me, the pinnacle of a lifelong passion for the art of Arthur Rackham – who illustrated *Peter Pan*, among other books – was a trip to see Kensington Gardens in London.

123. PRACTISE LOVINGKINDNESS

Buddha said, 'The thought manifests as the word. The word manifests as the deed. The deed develops into habit. The habit hardens into character. So watch thought and its ways with care, and let it spring from love born out of concern for all beings.'

This directive may be summed up in one word that is integral to the Buddhist spiritual tradition, 'lovingkindness', the practice of making a conscious and continuous effort to always treat others in a loving, kind and generous way – even those who have done you harm, and those whom you do not know and may never meet.

The real power of lovingkindness is that it is not just the recipients of your behaviour who benefit – you do, too. When you act with malice or greed, you become a smaller, meaner, less secure person; when you act with love, kindness, generosity of spirit and selflessness, you put yourself on a path towards becoming happier, more contented and more at peace with yourself and with others.

And no, it's not easy to do – nothing worthwhile ever is. Start small. For example, you might think that a neighbour at home with a small baby might be lonely and would appreciate a friendly chat, but habit or even shyness on your part means that you quickly make excuses, 'She's probably busy – and we won't have anything in common'.

Next time you have one of these thoughts, run with your first, generous impulse, and knock on her door with a bunch of flowers. The act of lovingkindness will resonate with the both of you for a long time to come.

124. BE MINDFUL

'Mindfulness' is another cornerstone of Buddhist philosophy. Put simply, it means becoming more conscious of what you say and do, and understanding the impact of your thoughts, words and deeds, however small.

Remaining calm and focused so that you can manage your responsibilities and take action throughout the day – and to enjoy your time on this planet and preserve your sanity – is a tricky business. The mindfulness technique is based on the idea that every act has three stages: before, during and after. Practise it when household clamour and clutter, kids and stressed-out spouses are raging all around you. Imagine yourself in the calm eye of a hurricane, poised and mindful despite the swirling chaos. Concentrate on breathing in the good, and breathing out the bad.

◆ **Before you do or say anything**, ask yourself, 'Will this benefit all beings?' If your heart says 'yes', do it. If it doesn't, then don't say or do something you may regret.

◆ **If you proceed** with the comment or act, ask yourself while you're doing it, 'Is this of benefit to all beings?' If the answer is still 'yes', continue; otherwise, stop.

◆ **When you have finished**, ask yourself for a final time, 'Was that of benefit to all beings?' Your heart may say 'yes' for a third time – or you may realise that, even though it seemed like the right thing to do while you were doing it, you would be better off not doing it again.

By continually checking in with yourself, you become more deliberate about what you do or say because you are aware of the consequences of your actions on yourself and on others. Your thinking simplifies; you reduce the whole situation to its simplest terms and basic principles.

Over time, practising mindfulness will become second nature and help you streamline your thoughts, making things clearer and easier.

125. ACCENTUATE THE POSITIVE

Newsflash: if you are suspicious, grumpy or angry, and you think that you are surrounded by negativity in general, you will be. If, on the other hand, you feel secure in yourself and aim to project your best qualities to the world, the more love, compassion and humour will be drawn to you.

Anaïs Nin wrote, 'We don't see things as they are; we see them as we are'. The more positive energy you give off, the more you'll receive. See the light, not the shade; look for what lifts you up, not what weighs you down.

If you're nowhere near a positive state of mind right now, these steps will help guide you there.

♦ **Thought-switch** Defining yourself in terms of negatives is an easy and insidious habit. If, for example, you have always regarded yourself as being shy and insecure, then that is exactly how you will present yourself to others, and they will react in ways that confirm your view. Next time you are faced with a situation where you have to speak to people you don't know, or attend a function that makes you nervous, boost your personal positivity meter up a few notches by saying to yourself, 'I may be shy, but that doesn't mean I'm insecure. I am secure in knowing I possess quiet strengths, such as my kindness and sincerity. I am going to focus on those characteristics and let them flow through me in everything I say and do'. If you hold your best characteristics in the front of your mind, other people will see them, too.

♦ **Avoid pessimists** Good health thrives on good company, just as misery and poor health also like company. Every family, school or office has the chronic complainers, the doom-and-gloomers, the gossips, the bitter and the foul-mouthed. These people will depress your mood and sour your attitude, tainting you with their negative life-view. Some may even be what psychologists call 'emotional vampires', people whose need to bring you down to their level verges on pathological because they 'feed' on your energy. Choose to walk, talk and be with enthusiastic, compassionate, content, encouraging people who restore your faith in human nature and help your spirit to grow. Regard these people as your 'positivity supplements' and take regular doses of them, just as you would vitamin supplements.

◆ **Send out heart energy** A Wiccan saying runs, 'There is no greater magic in the world than to join people together in love'. Just as you commit to regularly washing dishes and taking out rubbish, commit to using an emotional house-cleaning tool such as meditation, psychotherapy, writing and talking with friends to 'clean house'. This sweeps away negativity and prevents build-up of dark fears and grimy resentments, leaving your energy field free and clear to notice the sense of peace and harmony that constantly surrounds you, and to send out positive heart energy. The first step is to consciously notice something wonderful that is there for the taking: your son's smile, a tree covered in bright autumn leaves. Ask, 'Let this love flow into me'. Feel it slide into you and warm your heart, making you feel content and serene. Now push it gently away from you and let it spread outwards to others.

126. TAKE A GOOD LOOK AT YOURSELF

For many women and men, their personal power is defined by how they look. For example, a woman who grew up with the knowledge that her long blonde hair and long brown legs wielded a certain power can be unsettled when she wakes up middle-aged, with hair now short and brown, and legs marked with varicose veins, courtesy of three pregnancies.

Mourning the way you used to look – which has disappeared as surely as yesterday's rainbow – is depressing and futile. It can also make you feel trapped, because you think you need your looks to be happy. This is a rapid road to Stressville, the place where you go to spend more money trying to hang on to something that's gone. The women who equate being young with being desirable may also regard their sexual attractiveness in the same way: if they see themselves as having lost the power to influence others, it will spill over into how they rate their other talents, too.

Women are fantastically sexy, potent and gorgeous-looking at any age. Recognise that the way you used to look is just one way of defining who you are and how you relate to the world. Try this exercise.

◆ **Identify what you feel you must have in order to be attractive** – say, that you must have long, blonde hair or be ten kilos lighter. Ask yourself 'Is that really true?'

◆ **Entertain the possibility that it's not necessary** – you're just floating the idea, you don't have to believe it, you can still really, really want it to happen. But even the few moments of perspective you gain while imagining that it's not actually necessary for you to have long blonde hair or be much thinner can clear a way to looking forwards, not backwards.

◆ **Instead of thinking 'I've lost my looks'**, think 'I've outgrown *that* look'. The long, blonde hair might be gone, but the intelligence and humour in the eyes that you see in the mirror are a far more powerful ally.

127. REMEMBER, IT'S ALL LIFE

When Edward was small, he went through a stage where he refused to play with other children; he just wanted to sit by himself. He was perfectly happy about this, but I worried and felt guilty ('He's never going to cope in the real world'). My wonderful then-neighbour, a registered witch who wore floor-length turquoise scarves and kept three jet-black cats, taught me a great lesson when she said, 'He's just taking time out; let him be, it's all life'.

Life does not exist in a vacuum. Nor does it always run a certain way, or have a purpose – or at least not one that you can identify straight away. 'Everything that happens to you is your teacher,' said Mahatma Gandhi. 'The secret is to sit at the feet of your own life and be taught by it.' That means that kids like my Ed have got it right when they take time out to potter and mooch and mull quietly over the events of the day.

When you're small, it's easy to identify the things that distract you from this contemplative process: other people. However, when you're older, even if no one else is around, dozens of faceless demons and inner voices will rush to fill the void as soon as you create empty space. 'What are you doing? You're wasting time! You have no right to stop, not for even five minutes!' they cry.

Putting a name to these anxieties is the only way to prevent them from getting in the way of your chill-out time. And the name is guilt. Don't feel guilty about taking time out from being busy. Eat ice-cream for dinner. Talk to imaginary friends. Goof off, stare into space. Say – out loud, if you like, to the voices telling you that you're wasting time – 'I'm doing absolutely nothing, and I don't have to. I need time to think as well as time to do things. It's all life.'

It's only in these quiet moments that you become receptive and can tune in to the 'deep knowing' of what nourishes you, weed out what no longer works or doesn't feel right, and shift to make room for what does.

'Where does the body end and
the mind begin? Where does the
mind end and the spirit begin?'

B.K.S. Iyengar

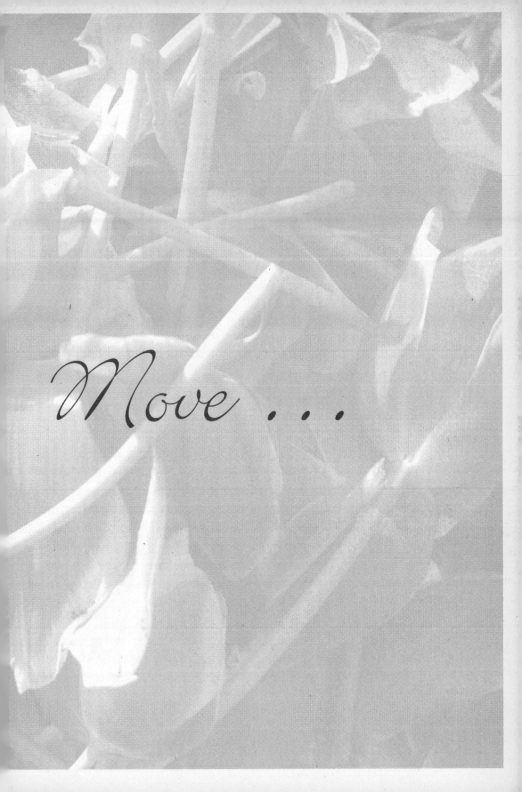

Move . . . .

While you're getting your mind into a calmer, more balanced state, don't forget to bring your body along for the ride. Make 'move–breathe–move' your daily mantra. Moving and breathing are the most basic ways you can take care of yourself – and they're also two of the main things you tend to stop doing when you're stressed and under pressure. Fitness isn't a gift for the fortunate few: it's a habit that you can learn to cultivate.

Exercise of any kind is a quick way to pep yourself up and get more energy, as well as an efficient method of burning off stress hormones and so encouraging you to slow you down and help you relax. Studies consistently indicate that exercise lifts your mood and keeps you feeling focused and 'on your game', as well as helping to keep you physically healthy. Researchers have found that people who exercise daily have lower stress levels than those who are sedentary. Exercise raises levels of brain chemicals called endorphins that help keep you feeling happy and peaceful. Sitting around, day after day, leads to a stagnant mind and a stiff body that's old before its time. A fit, supple body, on the other hand, goes hand in hand with a fit, supple mind.

Working out increases your heart and respiration rates, elevates your oxygen consumption and pumps up your metabolism. By increasing your capacity for tolerating physical stress in this way, you also deepen your capacity to cope with emotional stress. Push yourself beyond your comfort zone, whether on the weight bench or tossing a frisbee in the park, and you'll become stronger physically, and more stress-proof. On the pursuit of peace of mind, Charlotte Brontë wrote, 'It is not enough for humans to be surrounded by tranquillity. To find peace, one must have action'.

Exercise also gives you endurance and sustained energy, both of which are critical to coping with a stressful lifestyle. So bend, stretch, skip, hop, dance, run, swim, play, throw or jump. Don't wait to get sick before you decide to get up and start moving. You don't have to be at the gym or playing pro netball; if you're at the park with your kids, stretch really hard as you reach for that ball; if you're cleaning the house, pump it up as you sweep and polish.

Whether you're an exercise novice or you already have a regular routine, a series of daily stretching exercises is your most important first step.

Stretching helps to release tension stored in the body's muscles and improves flexibility, as well as boosting circulation, helping your body to eliminate waste more efficiently, and reducing the likelihood of injury during exercise. If you haven't exercised for a long while, start small: just a gentle ten-minute walk lifts your energy levels and invigorates mind and body. Choose a form of exercise that will fit easily into your routine, such as an early morning walk, or a twice-weekly aqua-dance class.

A good test to decide what type of exercise to do is to ask yourself, 'How do I want to feel afterwards?' If you're likely to be exercising after a stressful day, ask yourself whether you want to get rid of tension, perhaps with a vigorous kick-boxing session, or to wind down so you sleep soundly, which you are more likely to achieve with a mind–body regime, such as yoga or tai chi, both of which put the stress response in your body on hold so your body can regain its natural balance.

As your fitness level increases, try to vary the type of exercise you do. Learn tennis or golf, or take up a self-defence class. This will stop you from getting bored – which is the main reason why people give up exercise – and also make you use different muscle groups. Set realistic goals. When we form plans, we tend to overestimate our capacity to do something. Then, when we underachieve, we feel bad about ourselves. Set yourself up for success by making a reasonable commitment. For example, say you know you can easily walk three times a week for 20 minutes. Do this until it feels like little effort, then increase your time to 30 minutes, and so on. The more successful you are, the more your motivation grows.

128. EXERCISE YOUR FACE

If exercise can recondition your body, it stands to reason that it can also recondition your face. Along with the bone structure, there are fifty-five different muscles that make up your face and how you look. Although you may think your face gets plenty of exercise from constant speech and expression, in fact it is only getting exercise in the same directions, which does nothing for the facial muscles that are under-utilised, or for overall balance.

Facial exercises need not take long: 10–15 minutes daily will improve circulation and skin tone, help to relieve puffiness and de-kink stiff facial muscles. However, you must do them regularly. An on-and-off routine just won't achieve the desired effect. As with any exercise, the more you do it, the better the pay-off will be.

You'll find these exercises easier if you first apply a light coating of a good nourishing cream or a cold-pressed oil (e.g. almond oil) to lubricate the skin and protect against the forming of new lines. Wherever possible, do your facial exercises in a warm room or in the bath where the steam helps to relax the facial muscles.

◆ Lift your eyebrows and open your eyes wide. Open your mouth wide and say 'aaahhh' while sticking your tongue out. Hold for fifteen seconds.

◆ Think of your face as a clock. Starting with your chin, make the muscles of your face 'sweep' in a clockwise direction all the way from '6 o'clock' back to '6 o'clock'. Do the same thing counter-clockwise.

◆ To strengthen the mouth muscles, make an 'o' with your lips and then attempt to pull them together like a drawstring bag without actually letting them close. Reverse the action by trying to open your lips, but keeping them held tightly. Relax and repeat.

◆ Tilt your head backwards while lifting your chin to the ceiling. Hold this position while making chewing motions with the mouth.

◆ Slowly and gently roll your head around on your neck, as if trying to touch your shoulders with your ears. Do two rolls in each direction.

129. LOOK YOUNGER

Too much stress takes a toll not only on your mind and body, but on your looks as well, causing your skin to look aged beyond its years. This relaxing face and neck massage will stimulate circulation, release tension and make your skin more supple. Try it when the pressures of life are making you frazzled.

Before you start, make sure your hands, neck and face are clean. Rub your hands briskly together to generate warmth and energy, and apply a light nourishing cream or oil so you do not stretch or drag your skin. Your massage strokes should always work upwards.

◆ **Forehead** Place your fingertips on your temples and make large, slow circles. Then, using smooth strokes, run your fingers across your forehead, always moving away from an imaginary line down the middle of your face.

◆ **Cheeks and chin** Stroke along the sides of your nose, along your cheekbones to your ears. With the thumb and fingertips, gently pick up small sections of the skin with quick, light movements. Release a tense jaw by feeling along the jawbone and finding the indentation that is about an inch from where it's joined to the upper jaw, then massaging this point for a slow count of 30.

◆ **Ears and eyes** Gently lift your ears up, back and forwards in a circular motion. With the index finger of each hand, press the spot immediately behind the inner corners of your eyes. Press gently and firmly for a count of 5, then massage in tiny circles. Use your forefingers and thumbs to gently pinch along the bony ridge around your eyes, starting at the inner corners and working your way out and up along the brows.

◆ **Scalp** Spread your fingers through your hair and massage your scalp with small, circular movements. Use your thumbs to massage the hollows at the back of your neck where the spine and the skull join. Apply circular pressure for a slow count of 10, relax and repeat.

◆ **To finish**, lightly and rhythmically tap all over your face like raindrops, then press your temples gently.

130. REWARD YOUR HANDS

Your shoulders, arms and hands are your primary tools, and they work hard for you all day, whether they're lifting groceries, tapping away at a computer keyboard, cooking, cleaning or driving.

Look after them by regularly rubbing in a nourishing lotion or oil, taking regular breaks from repetitive work and stretching and shaking them. During any break, try these gentle stretches and massage moves.

◆ **Shoulders** Lift your shoulders up and breathe in. Breathe out, letting your shoulders drop and relax. Repeat 5 times. Support your left elbow with your right hand and, making a loose fist of your left hand, gently pound across your right shoulder. Using your thumbs and fingertips, make small circular movements to work more deeply into the muscles, moving from the back of your neck down your right shoulder. Repeat, using your right hand on the left-hand side of your body.

◆ **Arms** Straighten your right arm, open your palm and tap down the inside from the shoulder to the open hand using your left hand. Turn your arm over and tap up the back of your arm, from the hand to the shoulders. Repeat 5 times. Repeat on left arm.

◆ **Hands** Use your left thumb to work over your right hand, gently massaging the centre of your palm, then work the mound at the base of each thumb, pressing deep with your knuckles to release tension. Search out other sore spots and press with the thumb, holding for a count of 5. Carefully squeeze and massage the joints of each finger using your index finger and thumb. Pull out the fingers and briskly rub the fingertips to release any stress and tension in your hands. Repeat on the left hand.

131. SOOTHE YOUR FEET

Healthy, happy, pain-free feet mean a healthier body and a lighter, clearer mind.

Turn a simple footbath into an oasis of perfect peace by adding the benefits of reflexology. Reflexology is much more than just a foot massage; this ancient technique can have deeply balancing and healing effects. The theory is that every part of your body is mapped out on the feet: for example, the big toe relates to the head and brain, the lungs are spread across the ball of the foot, and the lower back is down near the heel. By massaging the relevant point on the foot, you can release tension and relieve blockages in the flow of energy to the corresponding part of your body.

This quick reflexology routine is easy to do at any time, and will help you to feel calmer and more focused.

◆ Empty a bag of marbles into the bottom of a footbath, and fill with enough warm water to come to just below your ankles. Add 5 drops of peppermint oil. The scent of peppermint helps improve cognitive ability and also has an invigorating effect on tired feet, putting some pep in your step. Roll your feet back and forward over the marbles to relieve stress and tension in your feet. Soak for 5 minutes to soften your skin and refresh your senses, then dry your feet thoroughly.

◆ Place your right foot on your left thigh and, using firm strokes, massage along the sole of your foot from toes to ankle. Using both thumbs, work with small, firm circles from the ankle to the toes, covering all of the sole. Inching your thumbs along, work all surfaces of each toe. Repeat this thumb-walking action across the ridge to where your toes meet the ball of your foot. Gently roll each toe between your thumb and forefinger, then give each toe a gentle tug.

◆ Bend your right knee and bring the heel in towards your right buttock. Starting from the instep, stroke both hands up the shin, and circle your knees. With your knee still bent, draw both hands up from your ankle and up the back of your leg.

◆ Stretch your leg out, flex and extend your toes, and do a few ankle rotations. Repeat on the left foot and lower leg.

132. BE CALM AND CENTRED

Here is a simple daily stretch that will start you on the road to discovering how your body works, and help you to develop inner calm, poise and balance. When you are ready, you can expand your repertoire of exercises, drawing on Pilates, tai chi, yoga and Swiss-ball routines.

◆ Stand with your feet shoulder-width apart, knees slightly bent and arms hanging loosely by your side. Inhale, straighten your legs and lift up one leg. Flex toes back towards you, then point them away; repeat 5 times. Rotate foot; repeat 5 times. Repeat with the other leg and foot.

◆ Turn arms outwards, inhale, and raise your arms so that the palms are facing each other over your head. Exhale and return arms to your sides; repeat 5 times. Raise your arms above your head again, this time stretching your left arm as high as you can while pulling down the right shoulder; repeat 5 times. Repeat on the other side.

◆ Bend your knees and turn arms inwards. Inhale and raise your arms to shoulder-height, exhaling as you bring your hands in front of your chest. Inhale, twist your upper body at the waist, first to the right, leading with the right arm. Return to the centre and exhale, then inhale as you repeat, twisting to the left, leading with the left arm. Return to the centre and exhale. Repeat 5 times.

◆ Straighten legs and step your right foot forward, bending your right knee and keeping your upper body straight and your weight evenly distributed over your hips. Feel the stretch along your inner thigh. Repeat on the other side.

133. CLEAR OUT THE COBWEBS

Your body's lymphatic system is a drainage system – if it isn't moving freely, it means that nobody's taking out the garbage.

Lymph is a clear fluid made up of protein, white blood cells and minerals. The circulation of this fluid around your body is critical to its ability to detoxify itself and regenerate tissue, and also helps to maintain a healthy immune system – the lymph also carries viruses and bacteria, eventually expelling them.

Your lymphatic system can be compromised by stress and fatigue. Try the following simple tips to help maintain lymph flow, speed up the removal of toxins from your body and strengthen your immune system.

◆ **Lymphatic massage** Position your hands at the centre of each clavicle (collarbone) and away from the centre of the neck. The fingers should be only slightly spread and pointing upwards. Applying gentle pressure, use the pads (not tips) of your fingers to sequentially press gently inward towards the middle of your body for 3 seconds, then outward for 3 seconds, moving like ocean waves upon the shore. Release for 3 seconds, then repeat 4 or more times. This will open the entire lymph system. Next, move to the temples. Place your fingers in the slight depression at the sides of your eyes. Using the same light pressure, draw the pads of your fingers back towards the tops of your ears. Perform 5 very light, gentle and slow strokes. Do this at least 2 more times.

◆ **Gently dry-brushing** your body before you shower removes dead skin cells, stimulates the lymphatic and circulatory systems, and promotes cell renewal. It is a super-stimulating early morning boost: your skin is full of nerve cells, and by stimulating the skin's surface you can wake up those cells and so wake up your whole body. Dry-brush at least two or three times a week to keep your skin rosy and glowing, and the tingling sensation it produces is invigorating as well. Before you step in the shower, use a natural bristle brush with a long handle or an exfoliating mitt to briskly brush every part of the body except the face and neck. Make long, sweeping strokes, always moving towards the heart. Brush from the hands to the shoulders, the feet up to the thighs, and the sides of the back towards the torso.

134. SAVE YOUR SPINE

'A flexible back makes for a long life,' says a Chinese proverb.

Long days on your feet running errands and locked into a static position in front of a desk make it difficult to maintain an upright posture. Maintaining core stability goes a long way towards preventing stiffness, increasing blood circulation and preventing back problems.

Perform this gentle, rolling-style move every hour or so. Use a rolling-pin, a rolled-up towel or a full bottle of water until you can do it without needing a prop.

◆ Stand with feet hip-width apart, knees bent. Hold the rolling-pin in both hands, flat against your breastbone, keeping your elbows bent.

◆ Inhale and bring your chin down towards your chest. Exhale and roll the rolling-pin down your body, rounding your shoulders and upper spine to follow its descent. Guide the rolling-pin down your tummy and legs, 'ironing' them straight and firm in your mind's eye.

◆ Straighten your arms as you approach the floor. When you can't go any lower, hang for a count of 5, looking down at the rolling-pin. Then, inhale and curl your body back up, using the rolling-pin as a guide to reverse the action.

◆ Repeat 3 to 5 times.

135. EASE SHOULDER STRAIN

Whole books have been devoted to tightening and toning butt muscles and reducing thigh size – this isn't one of them. Thighs, hips and bottoms are important, but strengthening your upper back and shoulders can make a significant difference to how you look and feel, especially to how relaxed you are. These muscles are not just responsible for holding you upright; they also open your heart centre and lift your chest and so make breathing easier. If your shoulders are underdeveloped, you'll end up with a rounded, slouched appearance, and an aching back as well.

Try this back-saving tip to become more aware of these forgotten muscles. You'll notice a dramatic difference in both your posture and performance. It's a subtle movement that rebalances your whole upper torso, facilitates ease of movement and engages deep muscles to improve stability and coordination. It's also mentally restorative, helping to reduce stress.

◆ When sitting or standing, don't pull your shoulders back.

◆ Instead, draw the bottom of your shoulder blades *down* and *in* towards your spine, while lifting your breastbone *up* and *outwards*. It may be uncomfortable at first, particularly if you're not accustomed to it, but get into the habit of holding your shoulders this way as it helps induce physical and mental relaxation.

◆ Hold the position for about 15 seconds. Add 15 to 30 seconds at a time until you're doing it without having to think about it.

136. COOL DOWN

One of the quickest and most effective ways to relax is to breathe slowly and calmly, letting the air fully inflate your diaphragm, right down to deep in your belly. However, most of us breathe much too quickly and shallowly, which means that the body takes in insufficient oxygen and retains tension. Learn the art of deep, diaphragmatic breathing and you can calm down anywhere and anytime, even if you have only two minutes to spare.

When you are first learning this technique, you may find it easier to lie down on the floor, as this helps you to focus attention on your breathing. Once you're familiar with it, you can practise it sitting, standing or while walking.

♦ Lie flat on the floor. Place a rolled-up towel under your neck so your airways are straight, but not tilting your head upwards. Rest your hands at the bottom of your rib cage, fingertips just touching.

♦ Breathe in through your nose for a slow count of 5. Focus on filling your lungs completely. Keep your shoulders still and focus on filling your chest and puffing out your abdominal cavity, using your fingertips as a guide to moving sideways and outwards, not scrunching up.

♦ Breathe out through your mouth for a slow count of 5, feeling your abdomen collapse and your stomach and chest muscles relax. Notice your shoulders: they should remain still; if you find they drop downwards, that means you lifted them towards your ears while inhaling. Be aware of this, and try not to do it with the next breath.

♦ Repeat 5–10 times until you have an even rhythm established. Try not to break between the in- and out-breaths, aim for a continuous flow of breath. On each out-breath, imagine all the tension leaving your body.

137. BALANCE YOUR BREATHING

The ancient yogis understood the connection between breath and power, believing the stomach area to be an important energy centre for the whole body. Yogic breathing techniques teach you to focus not just on breathing in, but on expelling as much air as possible so that inhaling is, in fact, the reflex action – not the other way around, which leads to shallow, inefficient breathing.

This energising exercise combines an easy spinal twist and breathing techniques to awaken your energy and soothe tense stomach muscles. It helps release physical and emotional tension, and can also provide relief for indigestion and cramps.

◆ Stand quietly, feet shoulder-width apart, and close your eyes. Lift your hands to your shoulders and touch them lightly, keeping elbows square to your sides.

◆ Breathe in, slowly twisting around to your left, keeping your back straight and eyes closed. Hold for a count of 3. Then exhale, twisting around to the right, and making a powerful 'ha!' or 'wooh!' sound to fully expel all the air in your lungs. Repeat, breathing in and slowly twisting to the right, then unwinding and exhaling to the left.

◆ Keeping your eyes closed, inhale, then allow your arms to fall loosely by your sides, and bend over, exhaling and making the loud 'ha!' sound as your upper body becomes limp and flops over. Your head should end up near your knees, your arms should swing downwards freely.

◆ Inhale deeply as you slowly rise back to the standing position, and open your eyes.

138. GAIN CONTROL

The Buddhist monk Thich Nhat Hanh wrote, 'Breathing in, I know that I am breathing in. Breathing out, I know that I am breathing out.'

In the Buddhist tradition, the breath is the foundation of all life; it is also a metaphor for the way you live your life. If you are often out of breath, or breathe poorly and shallowly because you are too busy with other functions, it follows that your fundamental connections with your inner self and with the world around you are also out of balance.

By becoming more aware of your breathing patterns, you tune in to your emotions. Learning to control your breath better through simple meditation exercises like the ones that follow help you to reduce blood pressure and calm your mind. Try them any time you need an instant escape from a hectic schedule – even three complete breaths can create a complete mood change.

◆ **Heartbeat breathing** Sit up straight, shoulders back, so you are not in a slouch. This opens your heart and makes it easier for you to notice your pulse. Close your eyes and begin to breathe rhythmically, in for a count of 4 heartbeats, out for a count of 4, then hold your breath for 4 heartbeats. Repeat 10 times. Increase your inhalation–exhalation-hold rhythm to 5 heartbeats for each step, then 6.

◆ **Tongue meditation** In classical yoga practice, the tongue is used to enhance the effects of the particular exercises or *asanas*. Clench your jaws for a count of 5; then release. Press your tongue against the roof of your mouth, as hard as you can, for a count of 5; then release. Stick your tongue out as far as it will go and – if circumstances permit – roar like a lion, opening your eyes wide. Repeat the exercise in reverse – roar, shut your eyes, press your tongue upwards, then clench your jaw, all for the count of 5. Finish with a yogic 'cooling breath': curl your tongue into a tube, letting the tip protrude slightly. Breathe in slowly and deeply through the space in your tongue, then breathe out the same way. Repeat.

◆ **Alternate nostril breathing** Straighten your spine, lift your chest forward, hold your head up and shut your eyes. Cover your left nostril with your left thumb and breathe in through your right nostril for a slow count of 10. Place your index finger over your right nostril and breathe out through your left for a slow count of 15 or longer. Visualise the breath coming in and up one side of your nose, then going smoothly down the other side in a continuous flowing movement. Repeat 10 times, lengthening the out-breath for an extra count each time.

139. RECHARGE YOUR BATTERIES

Some days are so hectic and stressful, emergency measures are needed. These three deep relaxation methods require no special equipment or training, all you need is the floor.

Placing yourself in a deeply relaxed state for even just 15 minutes two or three times a week is a powerful preventative measure against becoming over-stressed and overwhelmed. Deep relaxation also helps to speed up your cognitive processing abilities, and allows you to think more rationally.

Your body temperature will drop when you perform these exercises, so have a light rug handy.

◆ **Progressive relaxation** Lie down on the floor, close your eyes and focus on your breath. Breathe in deeply through your nose, and breathe out through your mouth. Focus on the feeling of your breath as it fills your abdomen, then as it falls when you exhale. Visualise all the tension leaving your body with each exhalation, bit by bit. Shift your attention to different parts of your body, beginning with your feet. Imagine your feet becoming so heavy that you couldn't possibly move them. Now shift your focus to your knees, then to your thighs and buttocks. Continue to shift your focus up your body, to your stomach, back, arms and head, seeing them becoming heavy and soft, and continuing to see tension dissolving and flowing away from your body with each out-breath. If you find your mind wandering, return your focus to your breath. Allow yourself to stay where you are for as long as you can. Being in a deeply relaxed state can alter your sense of time: you may feel as though half an hour has passed, when in fact you have been relaxing for just a few minutes. Give yourself time to return to your waking world. Only stand up when you feel ready.

◆ **Kitten curl** This exercise is simple yet deeply comforting because it helps you to collect your scattered energies, leaving you feeling stronger, more alert and better able to concentrate. Kneel on the floor, toes pointing behind you. Raise your arms straight upwards and inhale for the count of 5; then lie down, forehead touching the floor, eyes shut, with arms stretched out in front of you, palms facing downwards. Breathe out for a count of 10, feeling the stretch right through your shoulders and down towards the cervical and lumbar regions of your spine. Breathe in for a count of 5, then exhale for 10, sweeping your arms down past your sides, and turning the palms upwards. Clench your hands into tight fists for a count of 5, then relax for a count of 10, letting your hands fall open softly. Imagine that you are releasing negative energy and tension as your hands open. Repeat 10 times.

◆ **Block out noise** Even when you think it's quiet, your ears are besieged by sounds: the child next door crying furiously, a car outside honking its horn, a plane flying overhead. Sit cross-legged on the floor, spine straight, eyes closed and let your knees fall open loosely. (Lean against a wall if this is more comfortable.) Place your hands flat over your ears and press quite hard until you can't hear anything apart from the roar of your own blood – what you may have called 'the sound of the ocean' when you were a little child. Hold the pose for 2 minutes, breathing deeply and evenly. Slowly remove your hands and, using your thumbs and fingertips, carefully squeeze and tug on your earlobes, then pinch lightly all around the tops and edges of your ears. Rub your ears briskly, then open your eyes.

140. HAVE A BALL

Swiss exercise balls are large inflatable reinforced rubber balls that are available at some office supply stores, as well as from physiotherapists. Using one as part of a home-based exercise routine – or even instead of a desk chair at work – will boost your energy, tone your core muscles (especially your back and hips) and improve your balance. You may be sitting down, but don't be deceived; these simple moves will give you a good workout. If you haven't used a Swiss ball before, take the movements slowly.

♦ Sit slightly forward of the centre of the ball with the balls of your feet poised lightly on the floor, your hands touching the sides of the ball for balance. Begin with gentle seated bouncing to get the feel of the ball and feel the stretch in your thighs, then try pelvic tilts forward and back, followed by hip circles in first one direction, then the other (think of belly dancing).

♦ Kneel facing the ball, knees and feet together, hands flat on the ball and arms bent at the elbow. Roll the ball forwards a little way until your forearms are resting on top of the ball, contracting your stomach muscles to support your body as you hold the balance between your knees and the ball in a straight line for a count of 5. Then roll back.

♦ Lie on your back, arms straight by your sides and rest your legs together on the ball with your knees bent. Using your core muscles, push up your hips, leading with your pelvis, so your body forms a straight line from your shoulders to your toes. Tighten your bottom and stomach muscles, visualising them pulling in towards your spine. Hold for a count of 5, then release.

141. FREE YOUR CHI

The underlying philosophy behind traditional Chinese medicine is that good health revolves around the correctly balanced flow of *chi* (or qi), the subtle energy of the body. Chi flows around the body in channels called meridians, and along the meridians lie hundreds of points that link the various organs and functions of the body.

The Chinese view of life and health is enormously complex, but the concept of chi is relatively simple: it can be depleted or blocked or lost altogether through too much, too little or the wrong kind of food, drink, exercise, work, sex and emotions. It can also be restored, freed and increased if we look after ourselves correctly.

This classical sequence is said to increase the amount of chi in your body, with the side-effects of promoting mind–body balance and flexibility. It will help to loosen your joints and improve circulation, too, and is particularly helpful in a stressful work situation. Find a private spot, such as the bathroom, where you can do it for a couple of minutes.

◆ Stand easily, feet hip-width apart, arms by your sides. Starting with your legs and feet, simply shake out your body however you feel comfortable.

◆ Move up your body, shaking your hips, torso, arms and hands vigorously. Shake your head from side to side and up and down. Then move down your body again, shaking yourself freely as you go. Vigorously kick away all the stagnant energy that you've released from your joints and stiff areas.

◆ Finish by lifting your arms, taking a deep breath, then flopping over at the waist so your arms hang loosely, pumping your breath out with a loud 'ha!' Slowly swing from side to side to release tension, then slowly straighten up.

◆ Repeat as often as desired.

142. GROUND YOURSELF

Students of the Oriental martial arts, such as tai chi and aikido, are taught that true inner strength is not just about physical power; it's about being in harmony with yourself and your surroundings.

When you move mindfully – whether you are performing an exercise, playing sport, walking to the bus stop or simply bending over to pick up a shopping bag – you move with purpose. Critical to this is the concept of grounding yourself – of developing the feeling of being centred, poised and steadily connected with the earth at all times.

Perform this move any time during the day. Use it as a way of scanning yourself from head to toe to release tension and refocus body and mind. Deceptively simple because it is performed slowly, it is extremely good for relieving stress.

◆ Stand with your feet hip-width apart, knees gently bent, arms by your sides, eyes shut. Align your posture, concentrating on centring your body and ensuring that you are holding yourself evenly. Feel your weight settling down towards the earth, and concentrate on the idea of drawing up energy from the earth.

◆ Open your eyes, straighten your legs and rise up on the balls of your feet. Interlace your fingers and push your palms outwards and hold overhead for a count of 10.

◆ Now move into a shallow squat, knees softly bent and positioned over your toes, drawing your tailbone down towards the earth. As you enter the squat, allow your arms to float down to shoulder-height, palms facing down. Imagine they are absolutely weightless, that they are being held up by warm currents of air rising from the ground, not by your muscles. Visualise the earth's energy flowing up through your feet, your body and out through your fingertips, expelling negative forces.

◆ Return to the starting position and repeat 5 times.

143. SETTLE YOUR STOMACH

The Chinese words *chi nei tsang* translate as 'moving internal organs into balance'. It is also the name of a type of simple self-massage that aims to improve digestion and elimination by moving *chi* (energy) to your vital organs so that they work better.

Practitioners of traditional Chinese medicine believe that unprocessed emotions are stored in the digestive system, so on a more subtle level, this technique can help restore emotional balance by allowing your feelings to unfold and clarify.

◆ Lie on your back, legs hip-width apart, and place a pillow under your knees to keep them slightly bent.

◆ Place your hands on your stomach over your navel and inhale for a count of 10. Hold, then exhale for a count of 10. Repeat 5–10 times, until you feel calm and relaxed.

◆ When your belly area feels relaxed and neutral, breathe in deeply and imagine that you are drawing the breath right down towards your tailbone. Exhale, relaxing your jaw and allowing your mouth to fall open. Repeat, concentrating on the feel of your belly rising and falling under your fingertips.

◆ As you continue your breathing rhythm, start to massage your belly with your fingertips, moving out from the navel. Imagine that the flesh is full of knots and lumps, and use your fingertips to gently probe, knead and untangle them. When you find a sore or tender spot, hold your fingertips there and press firmly, breathing in and out as you do so.

◆ Continue working outwards with your fingertips until you get to your hip bones. Press the fingertips of both hands just inside the bones and lift upwards in a scooping motion towards the navel. At the same time, imagine you are gently lifting your internal organs, then settling them in a more comfortable, relaxed pattern than before.

◆ Repeat 5–10 times, or until your belly area loosens within.

144. REFRESH INSTANTLY

Yoga is a fantastic form of exercise, and it's suitable for men and women of all ages and all degrees of fitness. The precise postures are known as asanas, and they stimulate circulation, nourish your organs and soften muscles and ligaments. The deep stretches bring your skeletal and muscular systems back into balance, as well as making you more flexible. Yoga is a workout for the mind as well as the body.

This particular asana (Sarvangasana or Shoulder Stand) switches your nervous system 'off', leaving you feeling calm and in control. Your legs are elevated and the force of gravity is reversed, so blood and lymph that has pooled in your veins from prolonged sitting at a desk is drained back towards your heart. From a mental health perspective, this pose helps you to consciously stop, back up and regroup. It is also useful for tension headaches and fatigue.

♦ Lie on the floor with your buttocks pressed against a skirting board, and your legs pointing up, resting against the wall. If necessary, place a small pillow or rolled-up towel under your neck for comfort and support. Make sure that your body is at right angles to your legs, and that they are straight, not bent.

♦ Relax your arms and feet and close your eyes. Hold the pose for about 5 minutes.

♦ As an alternative position, you may like to spread your legs apart as far as they can go, and feel the stretch on the different muscles.

145. SQUEEZE TO SHIFT YOUR MOOD

Simple isometric exercises can help to reduce blood pressure, boost circulation and improve the flexibility of muscles and ligaments. The repetitive actions are also soothing to the mind, helping to release tension while acting as a focal point for a mini-meditation that you can do any time, anywhere: at your desk, in the car or even while standing at the sink brushing your teeth.

◆ **Hands** Hold tightly to the arm-rests of your chair, the edge of your desk or the kitchen bench or the steering wheel if you're waiting in traffic. Squeeze as tightly as you can for a count of 5. Repeat 5 times, then shake hands vigorously.

◆ **Feet** Kick off your shoes and use your toes to pick up a pencil or a marble. Squeeze as hard as you can for a count of 5, then release. Repeat 5 times. Another idea is to keep a foam toe separator (used for pedicures and sold at pharmacies or salons) in your desk drawer. When you feel the tension rising, slide it between your toes (you can use it even if you're wearing pantyhose) and clench it tightly.

◆ **Gut** A quick way to slow down is to focus on parts of your body, such as your belly and – excuse me – your bum. Suck in your stomach and squeeze your anal and pelvic floor muscles as you inhale and hold for a count of 10. Exhale, release the muscles, and feel the relaxed, warm sensation.

146. JUMPSTART YOUR BODY

Unlike many fitness activities, yoga is not goal-driven. It's not about who wins, who finishes first, who performs best or who has the most perfectly toned figure. Yoga is primarily about practice. This is a difficult concept for many Westerners to grasp at first, because we rarely practise something just for its own sake. Yoga's spiritual approach is refreshing in a too fast world, because it offers a refuge from competitive-style approaches to fitness and health. The idea is to open yourself to the experience without worrying about what you do or do not manage to achieve. It's about taking a more measured approach, discovering the subtleties of skeletal alignment and exploring your body's abilities and limitations. It's also about learning the mental discipline of accepting things the way they are and not becoming too attached to an outcome, which is a powerful tool for facing the everyday stresses of life.

The Sun Salutation is a classic exercise for releasing stress and tension. It's also the perfect way to kickstart your day, because it massages every organ in your body as well as stretching every muscle. It should be carried out slowly and while observing the suggested breathing. Concentrate on your breath. Breathe in fully as you stretch upwards, and breathe out fully as you bend.

♦ Stand with your feet together, palms in a prayer position. Breathe in and raise both hands above your head, bending slightly backwards from the waist, and tilting your head back. (Position 1)

♦ Breathe out and slowly bring your upper body forward and down, bending from the waist. Place your hands flat on the floor on either side of your feet. Bend your knees if necessary. (Position 2)

♦ Breathe in and slide your right foot backwards, lowering your right knee to the floor to balance yourself. Look up and arch your back gently, keeping your hips low and as straight as possible.

♦ Breathe out and slide your left foot back as well, taking the weight of your body on your hands and toes, keeping your back and arms straight.

- Keeping your toes curled, move your bottom back towards your heels. Breathe out and move your chest along the floor, moving from front to back keeping your hips and bottom pointing up. Only your toes, knees, hands, chest and forehead should touch the floor.

- Breathe in and drop your hips towards the ground, keeping your legs together and the soles of your feet pointing upwards, your back arched and head facing up, pushing until your arms are straight.

- Breathe in as you curl your toes under and point your bottom upwards, creating an inverted 'v' shape. Your heels should be flat on the floor, your head dropped gently forward.

- Breathe in and slide your left foot backwards, dropping your left knee to the floor. Exhale and bring your right foot forward as you bend at the waist, forward and down.

- Breathe in and lift both arms above your head. Breathe out and lower your arms, bringing your palms together in the prayer position to finish.

- Exhale and move back into position 2, bending forwards, placing your hands flat on the floor beside your feet.

- Return to position 1, standing with feet together, hands in prayer position.

147. EASE EYE STRAIN

The Bates method is a series of exercises that aims to 're-educate' the eye muscles and improve eyesight. The exercises provide easy and soothing two-minute time-outs throughout the day, helping you to get a fresh perspective on what you're doing. They are especially helpful when your eyes are tired from spending too long in front of an unforgiving computer screen, particularly in an air-conditioned or centrally heated office.

◆ Every morning, close your eyes and splash them 20 times with warm water, then 20 times with cold. At bedtime, repeat the exercise.

◆ Throughout the day, blink frequently, about 15 times per minute.

◆ Cover your eyes with your palms to rest them completely 3–4 times a day. Listening to music will help you relax even further.

◆ Hold your forefinger 15–25 cm (6–10 in) from your eyes and focus on it. Move the finger from your left shoulder to the right, and follow with your eyes. Do this at least once a day.

◆ Do the same exercise, but focus on the moving background instead.

148. RESTORE AND REVITALISE

All yoga postures are superb for improving your balance, concentration and coordination. The Downward-facing Dog is almost a complete practice session in itself. It helps strengthen your arms and legs, aligns your spine into its optimum position, encourages deep breathing by opening the chest area, aids digestion and circulation, and is also deeply calming for the mind.

Use it to power up your mind, body and spirit when you feel drained and exhausted.

- Start on your hands and knees, wrists directly under the shoulders, knees directly under the hips. Breathe in and lift yourself up, straightening arms and legs and lifting your tailbone to create an inverted 'v' with your body. Tuck your chin in slightly towards your chest and align your head and neck with your arms. Hold for a count of 5.

- Exhale, pressing your hips down and back, keeping your arms and legs straight and balancing your weight on the balls of your feet and the palms of your hands. Lift your chest and draw your shoulders back. Hold for a count of 5.

- Repeat 5 times.

149. GO FOR A SPIN

Developed as a meditative practice thousands of years ago in Turkey, the practice of spinning was passed down from generation to generation by spiritual seekers known as 'whirling dervishes'. The flowing, whirling movement of spinning around in circles is thought to boost energy and focus the mind simultaneously. Spinning also helps improve balance and coordination.

◆ Stand with feet hip-width apart, arms straight out at shoulder-height. Keep your knees and shoulders soft.

◆ Start to spin clockwise on the spot; go as fast as you can but don't race. If you feel giddy, slow down and perform the spin slowly and carefully, in a controlled manner. You should feel a gentle lifting of your senses, not out of control. Prevent dizziness by returning your gaze to a single point with every circle that you make.

◆ Repeat 3–5 times, then stop and stand still with your hands in a prayer position until you feel stable. Breathe in, raise your arms over your head and look up. Then exhale, bringing your arms down to your sides.

150. INTEGRATE BODY AND MIND

All forms of exercise will help you to feel fitter and more supple. But when thinking about ways to improve your fitness, coordination exercises don't spring readily to mind. Yet we could all feel a lot better in body and mind if we paid more attention to developing our rhythm, poise and posture.

As a child, you would have been ideally balanced and fluid in your movements. Yet as time passes and you've adapted yourself to a stressful life, you lose that easy freedom of movement and unconsciously acquire patterns of movement that work against your body's abilities, resulting in tension and rigidity.

This particular exercise features integrative movements that help develop balance in the brain as well as the body. It involves moving your arms and legs in opposition across the body's midline.

◆ Stand in front of a mirror, feet hip-width apart and arms hanging straight down your sides.

◆ Raise your left knee up to your chest; at the same time, move your right hand across the middle of your body to rest your hand on the outside of your left knee. Swing your left arm out to the side for balance.

◆ Return to the starting position, and repeat with the left hand and right knee. Repeat 10 times on each side. Aim to establish a brisk rhythm, like a metronome, to build momentum and balance.

151. SWING YOUR HIPS

Pilates exercises are popular in gyms and dance studios around the world. Unlike aerobics or pump classes, they are performed at a leisurely pace; the movements are flowing and controlled with specific breathing patterns to improve coordination and muscle stamina.

This slow, easy, comforting Pilates exercise is excellent for getting the circulation of blood and lymph going again in your lower back and buttocks, and helps promote deep, effective breathing. It's superb when performed at the beginning of the day to get you focused, and at the end of the day to empty the lungs of stale air and relieve cramps or stiffness after sitting or standing for long periods.

◆ Place a mat on the floor, or fold a large towel or blanket lengthwise and place that on the floor. Lie on it on your back, feet slightly apart, arms up over your head. Press your spine as flat to the floor as you can.

◆ Breathe in and, at the same time, lift your feet and roll your knees up towards your chest. Hold the front of your shins firmly with your hands, tighten your tummy muscles, tuck your chin in and round your lower back to push the stretch as far as is comfortable for you.

◆ Staying rounded like a little ball, rock back and forth slowly on your back. Breathe in as you rock backwards and breathe out as your rock upwards. Avoid rocking on your neck.

◆ Repeat 5 times.

152. STRETCH LIKE A CAT

This rhythmic exercise is excellent for the lungs and breathing because it opens your chest, stretches the front of your shoulders and torso, and unlocks the tension that gets lodged in your neck and lower back. It is superb when performed first thing in the morning because it expels stale air from the lungs after sleeping. It's very beneficial for backache.

♦ Kneel on your hands and knees, aligning the wrists directly under the shoulders. Keep the knees apart, directly under hips.

♦ Pull your stomach muscles in and curve your spine up.

♦ Breathe in and lift your belly up and in towards your spine so that your back and neck are relaxed and elongated. Breathe out as you arch your back upwards as fully as is comfortable, dropping your head towards the floor and tucking your tailbone under.

♦ Breathe in and reverse the movement, lifting your tailbone, drawing your shoulders back, and pushing your chest forward so your back softens and your stomach sinks towards the floor.

♦ Repeat 5 times. Visualise the smooth, supple stretches of a cat, and aim for the same flowing movement between each sequence.

153. STAND TALL

Holistic healers refer to energy fields around our bodies. When we're stressed, the energy tends to free-float around our heads, making us feel unstable and off-centre.

This gentle yoga posture helps maintain mental equilibrium and develops your balance and flexibility, keeping you supple, which is important for an all-round feeling of relaxation. I find it is excellent for cooling down – both physically and mentally – and for refocusing energy. When you feel centred and grounded, it's not so easy for other people's attitudes and behaviour to knock you over.

To help you find your balance when you start, place one hand on a wall for support. This exercise should be done with bare feet. If you're at work, kick off your shoes.

◆ Stand up tall and straight with your feet slightly apart and parallel, with toes spread. Fix your eyes on something in the middle distance. Breathe naturally and evenly, and concentrate on balancing your weight evenly between your feet.

◆ Lift your right foot and place the heel against the inner side of your left thigh, with your toes pointing down. Use your hand to keep it there if you like. Keep looking at the point in the middle distance to help keep your balance.

◆ Bring your hands together in a prayer position. Breathe in and out 3–5 times. Now stretch your arms out to the sides at shoulder height. Breathe in and out 3–5 times. Raise your arms in a wide, open gesture towards the ceiling. Keep focusing on the point in front of you. Think about the strength and poise of a tree, how its roots are firmly locked into the soil, how its branches spread towards heaven. Think of yourself as strong and grounded, yet flexible and relaxed enough to sway in an imaginary breeze and let the wind play in your hair. Hold the position for a count of 10, then repeat on the other side.

154. STAMP LIKE A DRAGON

Chi gung (or *qi gong*) is a wonderful holistic mind–body exercise, meaning it exercises the body, mind and emotions.

This exercise combines deep breathing techniques with precise movements and mental concentration. It is a simple but effective way of relieving tension, and boosts energy levels by expelling stale, negative energy. It also improves concentration and even increases creativity by forcing you to concentrate on what you're doing.

Practise it first thing in the morning and throughout the day whenever the opportunity presents itself. Aim for a smooth, gentle movement. Take your time and enjoy the strengthening, steadying sensation that it brings.

- Stand comfortably, feet hip-width apart, arms by your sides. Close your eyes.

- Breathe out, rising slowly on your toes as high as you can and stretching your fingers down towards the floor as hard as you can at the same time. Hold for a count of 5.

- Breathe in and return your heels slowly to the ground, relaxing your arms as you do so. Open your eyes and stamp first one foot, then the other.

- Repeat 5 times.

155. SHAKE YOUR TAIL FEATHER

We've all been guilty of sitting in our chair for just those few minutes too long as we try to finish something off, only to grapple with cramp and lower back pain as a result. Quickly release tension in your lower back with this gentle two-minute rotation.

◆ Stand up and step back from your desk.

◆ Place your feet hip-width apart and bend your knees slightly. Place your hands on your thighs.

◆ Bend forward from the hips, keeping your back straight.

◆ Sway your torso gently to the left while stretching your hips and buttocks up and out to the right.

◆ Return to the starting position and repeat. Aim to move smoothly from one side to another, so your body moves like a pendulum.

156. HANG LOOSE

Stretching restores mobility and releases a good deal of stress. Stretching before and after exercise will help protect your muscles and reduce your chances of injury. It will also improve your posture and you will be far less likely to suffer from neck, shoulder and back pain.

This easy stretch is subtle but effective. It is based on classical yoga moves that boost adrenal and digestive function, and will give you an energy boost. It's also a great instant time-out, even if you have only two minutes to calm down and put some distance between stressful meetings or until the kids come home from school. It should feel pleasurable and liberating. Don't hurt your back by over-reaching or pushing too hard.

◆ Stand with your feet hip-width apart, toes pointing straight ahead.

◆ Clasp elbows with opposite hands, breathe in and take your arms over your head.

◆ Exhale and bend forward from your hips until you feel tension in your hamstrings, keeping your back straight. Visualise your muscle fibres elongating and relaxing. Bring your hips and chest as close to your legs as possible. As you hang there, you'll feel your lower back and neck muscles begin to stretch and soften, too.

◆ Release your elbows and let your hands flop to the floor.

◆ Inhale, rolling slowly upwards, to the count of 10, finishing in a slight back-bend with hands clasped behind your back at the base of your spine. Hold for a final count of 10, breathing normally, then straighten.

157. STIMULATE THE DANTIEN

In Chinese *chi gong*, the *dantien* (a point approximately three finger-widths above your navel) is regarded as the storehouse of chi (*qi*), your body's energy. This exercise is also good for your lower back muscles, stimulates the circulation of blood and lymph, and elevates your mood.

◆ Sit against a wall with your back straight. Angle your pelvis forward (sit on the edge of a folded towel if you wish).

◆ Bend your knees and slide your legs towards you as you breathe in, then let your knees flop out to the sides and bring the soles of your feet together; breathe out.

◆ Breathe in, and draw your heels as far back towards your pubic bone as is comfortable, keeping the outer edges of your feet on the floor; breathe out.

◆ Close your eyes and visualise your spine lengthening upwards, leading with an invisible string coming from the top of your head.

◆ Bring your right hand towards your stomach and hold it there, palm-side down. This is where the *dantien*, your energy source, is located.

◆ Place your left hand over your right, and concentrate on your *dantien*. Breathe in for a count of 5, feeling the breath flow into your abdomen as you do so, and make gentle clockwise circles with your hands. Breathe out.

◆ Continue for 3–5 minutes.

158. BALANCE YOUR ENERGY

First recorded in osteopathic literature in the 1930s, the practice of shifting energy within the body by the power of intention was used to help speed post-surgical recovery and ease pain. It is also much used in alternative treatments for cancer and other degenerative diseases, as a means of focusing the body's ability to rebalance and heal itself.

Energy balancing is based on the idea of 'intending' – or imagining – that healing energy radiates from your hands, and that you can direct it towards any part of your body. Energy redirection is particularly helpful for parts of the body that bear the brunt of a stressful lifestyle, such as the lower back and neck.

Use this technique on yourself, a co-worker, child or partner.

◆ Close your eyes and place your hands lightly together, fingertips and thumbs just touching. Visualise warm, bright rays of energy flowing evenly back and forth between your fingertips.

◆ Keeping your fingertips together and holding the idea of the healing rays in your mind's eye, concentrate on the injured or sore area you wish to heal.

◆ Lightly place one hand on top of the area and the other underneath (or in the front and back). Imagine that the healing rays are still flowing between your fingertips, now passing through the painful spot, warming and healing it. Think of your hands as jumper cables, and the tissue or body area in the middle as a flat battery that you are recharging with energy.

◆ Continue for 3–5 minutes, shifting your hands slightly so that the energy is distributed evenly.

◆ Bring your hands back together and fold them lightly, then open your eyes.

159. JUMP FOR JOY

Researchers at England's Nottingham University have found that women who jump or skip rope on the spot fifty times a day live longer than those who don't. In this study, women who performed this quick and easy exercise reported having much more energy. Bone scans have shown that, over time, skipping helped strengthen bones.

Skipping is an aerobic exercise, meaning it strengthens the heart and lungs, as well as a strength-training one that builds muscle and improves bone density, helping to ward off osteoporosis. It's also a quick way to beat stress. For one thing, it's fun: it's almost impossible to brood on dark thoughts and problems when you're jumping up and down – your body's endorphins (natural mood-lifting chemicals) kick in automatically. And for another, it is mentally and physically absorbing, forcing you to concentrate on coordinating your movements and focusing your attention on the rope and your jumping rhythm.

Skipping is a great way to warm up and will stimulate the circulation of blood and lymph, helping to expel toxins and stale air. Buy a skipping rope from a toy shop or fitness equipment store. If you haven't skipped since you were small, these steps will refresh your memory.

- Stand with your feet side by side. Hold the ends of the skipping rope and let the rope fall behind your heels.

- Bring the rope forward, over your head, in one even movement and hop as you twirl it towards you, giving a little jump at the same time so it passes behind you again.

- Repeat, building up speed as you establish a rhythm.

160. LEARN SELF-DEFENCE

My friend Lorraine talked me into taking a self-defence class a couple of years back. Apart from a nagging feeling that I 'should' learn these skills to protect myself against city predators, I had never really been interested, and I was concerned that I would need to be much stronger and fitter than I actually was.

I was pleasantly surprised to find that none of the exercises required strength or speed. I discovered that simple tricks could save your life, such as making a noise and jabbing vulnerable spots. I was also taught to try anything to get rid of an attacker – slap, scratch, kick, scream. As I role-played fending off an assailant, I caught sight of myself in the full-length mirror. For a moment, I didn't recognise the wild-eyed woman yelling, ducking and kneeing a man nearly twice her size in the groin. Then I realised that this class had had an unexpected and liberating benefit – it had given me confidence to try things that felt right for me.

Most of the time, when thinking about ways we can improve our fitness and embark upon an exercise program, we are caught somewhere between feeling confident about getting started, and feeling worried about failing at it. Sir Winston Churchill said, 'Never give up – never give up – never give up.' Learning self-defence is one way of building your personal power, giving you self-belief and the determination to keep on going and turn things around, no matter how many times someone tries to get in your way. Have the courage and confidence to do something new, and grow from the experience. Taking risks often brings great rewards.

161. GET UP AND BOOGIE

In spite of a dodgy ankle and an even more uncertain sense of rhythm, I have found nothing that gives me such a feeling of exhilaration and renewed optimism as dancing. My favourite time to dance is when I'm doing housework – a little moonwalk here, a little tango there, followed by dazzling disco queen moves and an air guitar solo, complete with jutting hips and pained expression. Of course, Edward and Randall regard this habit with undisguised horror: 'You don't seriously mean they used to dance like that? Gross!'

Dancing is one of the simplest, yet most effective ways of relaxing your body and mind and recharging your spirit. For centuries, native cultures have understood that dancing is a form of moving meditation, and people have used it as a way of communicating altered states of consciousness.

There are dozens of different dance classes on offer, and each will create a different sort of mood, as well as help to improve your fitness and give you some fun. If, for example, you want to feel more physically empowered, sign up for tango or ceroc classes. If you feel like getting in touch with your cultural roots, then everything from belly dancing to bootscootin' is available. If you just want to kick up your heels, try learning the twist or the Charleston. It only takes a few minutes to find a class: surf the Web, or call your local YWCA or council. Don't be shy, and don't worry about what other class members will think.

If a class doesn't appeal, you can still use dance at home as a form of easing physical and mental stress, reconnecting with your senses and simply celebrating the joy of being alive. You don't need training, but you do need music. Studies show that people who work out to music, either by themselves or in classes, have significant increases in cognitive function, especially in the parts of the brain that handle abstract thought and creativity. So, choose music that you enjoy and which inspires you to move energetically, sensuously and joyously. Push back the furniture so you've got room to move.

If you feel self-conscious or stiff, get yourself moving with this easy, rhythmic exercise. It will strengthen and tone your legs and thighs, loosen up your hips and make you feel more sure on your feet, as well as give you a sense of gathering energy.

- Stand with your feet hip-width apart, hands hanging loosely by your sides.

- Swing your arms up above your head, at the same time as you take a step back with your left foot and land on your toes. Feel equally balanced on both feet. Hold for a moment, then bring your left foot back, your arms down and clap your hands together. Repeat on the other side.

- Next, perform the same move, this time lunging sideways to the right – then the left, continuing to swing, bounce, bop and clap. Repeat.

162. GET UP, GO OUT, START WALKING

When was the last time you went for a walk? If you can put one foot in front of the other, you can walk. Henry David Thoreau wrote that, 'An early morning walk is a blessing for the whole day.' The world's easiest and cheapest exercise also helps you to calm down, lose weight and prevents disease.

Walking has no prerequisite in terms of fitness level; all you need is time. It's also weatherproof – just throw on a slicker and old runners, and splash your way through the puddles. However, these tips can improve your potential to reap toning and metabolic benefits.

♦ Take normal length strides – don't over-stride. Ensure a strong upward lift on the ankle of the leading foot as it moves to the heel strike. Push off well each time – feel the power and rhythm this gives you.

♦ Swing your arms naturally backwards and forwards, in opposition to your legs. Keep them slightly bent and close to your sides; your leading arm should not go too high.

♦ Increase speed and intensity if you wish by bending your elbows at a 90-degree angle by your sides, forearms parallel and hands in loose fists. As you walk, drive the elbows back and behind you, then back up to rib-cage level; this will propel you forward at a faster pace.

♦ Don't lean forwards or backwards. Leaning forwards and keeping your eyes on the ground is bad for your posture; leaning backwards can affect the stability of your pelvis, and shorten your stride. Actively think about keeping your torso erect, and keeping shoulders and hips square as you walk.

♦ Don't swing your arms across your body's midline as you stride; this can slow you down and affect your walking rhythm as well, causing you to rotate your torso and sway your hips. Do keep your arms pumping forward and back alongside your torso.

163. THROW SOMETHING

You don't have to be sporty or athletic to play simple toss-and-catch games with others or by yourself. They're not strenuous, but they do force you to learn patience and determination, and to focus on what you are doing. They also get you moving, keep your hands fit and supple, release pent-up aggression and develop good eye–hand coordination, which keeps you mentally alert. And they're fun. You don't even have to keep score.

Try these easy favourites.

◆ **Darts** A very effective way of getting out of a bad mood especially if you imagine you are spearing a particular problem with some force and 'killing' it. Set up a dartboard on the back of a door in the house or inside a garage or cellar. (Remember that darts are potentially dangerous, and safety precautions should be exercised, especially if children are around.)

◆ **Horseshoes** Horseshoe pitching sets, comprising four or six metal horseshoes and two stakes (to be hammered into the ground, which is also great for getting rid of stress) are available from toy and hobby stores. Toss those horseshoes over and over again.

◆ **Basketballs** Mark throwing lines on the driveway with chalk if you feel like a challenge. Dribble the ball, try new angles and variations on the simple throw, such as throwing the ball sideways over your head with one arm, holding both hands over your head and throwing the ball forward, or facing away from the hoop and throwing the ball backwards.

◆ **Frisbees** Said to be named for Elihu Frisbee, a college student who, in 1827, rebelled against compulsory chapel attendance by throwing the collection plate across the campus grounds, thus giving rise to the flying discs seen in parks ever since. Frisbees come in a wide variety of colours and sizes – some even glow in the dark – and they are a great way to get some exhilarating, silly fun. Tossing a frisbee gets you out and about in the fresh air, perhaps with a dog or a child for company. As a bonus, the common forms of frisbee-tossing – the underhand delivery and the backhand throw – help loosen and stretch wrists that have been clamped over a computer keyboard for too long.

164. BOUNCE ON A TRAMPOLINE

Trampolining is one of the fastest growing competitive sports in the world. Trampolines have also been installed in schools and universities and military-training establishments because of their stress-reducing prowess. Even simple bouncing up and down teaches you coordination, balance and control.

A trampoline in the backyard will provide a great spot to burn off tension.

No backyard? Buy a mini-rebounder from a department store or sporting goods supplier. Hop on and stand with your feet together, hands by your sides. Start with small jumps, raising your arms out to the side to form jumping jacks. Once you've got your rhythm going, clap your hands together over your head, alternate from one foot to another, or twist back and forth. Bounce your blues away.

165. LIGHTEN YOUR LOAD

When thinking about your fitness and ways to improve your overall wellbeing, think about the stuff you carry with you every day: handbags, groceries, briefcases, backpacks, nappy bags, iPods, rucksacks. Carrying heavy bags will play havoc with your posture and your ability to move freely and set you on the path to neck and shoulder injuries.

Here are the main culprits to avoid.

- **Shoulder bags** Swap to a backpack or bum-bag, if possible, where the weight is distributed evenly on your back. If that's not possible, at least choose a shoulder bag with a cushioned strap and keep shifting sides when carrying it. Clear out any heavy and unnecessary items, including layers of ancient tissues, receipts and wrappers.

- **Shopping bags** Never pick up anything by twisting or bending or reaching awkwardly. Bend your knees, distribute your weight evenly on both feet, and use your full body strength. When carrying loads, try to distribute the weight evenly in both hands.

- **Telephones** Never hold the phone between your ear and shoulder while doing something else with your hands. Use a headset or earpiece. During phone calls, stand up and walk, step side to side, do knee lifts or stretch.

166. WORK OUT AT YOUR DESK

The best fitness tips aren't always to be found at the gym or even outside in the fresh air. The most important thing you can do to help you relax and stay fit is simply to keep moving, even when you're stuck at your desk.

◆ **Massage your hands** Keep a tube of cream at your desk and give yourself a soothing hand massage. Search out sore spots, press with your thumbs, and hold for 10 seconds. Finish by making tight fists and doing several quick air-punches, then shaking them out and rolling them in wide circles.

◆ **Tame shoulder tension** 'Walk' your right fingertips along your left shoulder, applying firm pressure wherever muscles are tight. Repeat on the right shoulder.

◆ **Play footsie** Keep a golfball on the floor under your desk. Take your shoes off while sitting and roll the sole of each foot firmly over it.

◆ **Thump your thighs** Lightly pound the insides and outsides of your arms and legs with your knuckles. This stimulates circulation and boosts your mood.

◆ **Pull faces** When no one is looking, smile. Raise your eyebrows and lower them a few times. Open your mouth and stick out your tongue, as far as you can. Place your tongue against the roof of your mouth and press it as hard as you can, then release.

◆ **Buy a back massager** These roller-style wooden massagers are wonderfully relaxing. Keep one in your desk drawer and use it to ease muscular tension in your neck and back.

◆ **Joggle on the spot** Stand up and do a joggle – a cross between a quick jog-on-the-spot and a shake. Then move on to the next task, refreshed.

◆ **Keep a yo-yo** in your drawer to help relieve tension and relax hands and wrists.

◆ **Stretch your legs, even if you're sitting down** This quick stretch will help you to sit comfortably for longer. Cross your legs, placing your right ankle above your left knee. Gently push your right knee down, so that you feel a stretch in your right hip. Take your time in the stretch, feeling the pull in your hip and buttock. Repeat on the other side.

◆ **Let off steam** If you're angry and overwhelmed, just get up from your desk and rush up a flight of stairs. Anger produces energy that needs to go somewhere, and running it off helps to rebalance you. Walk down slowly, feeling the sole of each foot as it touches the ground. Even the most upsetting situation will look better when you have shocked your system with sudden movement, rather than just sitting still and fuming on the inside.

◆ **Get out of that chair** Turn a 10-minute walk at lunchtime into a powerful moving meditation by repeating an affirmation, such as 'I am moving forward, one step at a time' or just counting steps. Count the first 5 steps in your head. At the sixth, begin at 1 again, and count to 6. With the seventh, begin at 1 again, and count up to 7. Continue the pattern of walking and counting until you reach 10. Then begin all over again.

167. DRIVE A CALM CAR

Turn your car into a place to find solitude and calm away from home. Keep it reasonably clean and clutter-free, and protect yourself against in-car pollution by minimising driving during peak hour. Heavy traffic elevates concentrations of pollutants like carbon monoxide and benzene inside your car. Prolonged exposure to these may cause variations in heart rate and an increase in blood-clotting problems. Although these changes are reversible and unlikely to pose an immediate threat to healthy travellers, they may raise the risk of heart attacks and strokes in people with existing health problems.

When you're on the road, keep your distance from other cars and trucks. For added protection, invest in a high-efficiency particle (HEPA) filter, which may help reduce particle concentrations in indoor air.

Here are some other tips to turn your car into an on-road sanctuary.

♦ Place a flower or a favourite photograph on the dashboard.

♦ Stock it with bottled water and a selection of healthy, energising snacks, e.g. trail mix or a fruit-and-nut bar.

♦ Wipe down the dashboard, steering wheel and upholstery regularly with a relaxing essential oil, such as lavender or ylang ylang.

♦ Make the 'om' sound, up and down the scale, when you're driving. It's very calming, and no one will be able to see that you're doing it. Experiment with a simple, positive mantra while you're driving to focus your thoughts and counter frustration, e.g. 'Ommm … let me breathe deeply and fully'. 'Ommmm … let me enjoy this day and smile often.'

♦ The type of music you listen to when you're driving should create the type of mood you want to experience. Do you want to feel upbeat and excited? Or relaxed and quiet? Sing along as loudly as you like, and don't hold anything back. Whoop, whistle, hum, smile and play a bongo beat on the steering wheel. Noise-making is a safe means of releasing feelings that otherwise might explode in a much worse form later on. Your tension will turn to a smile.

♦ Get road rage under control: unless there is danger, don't honk your horn. If you're stuck in traffic, do something else to take your mind off the situation, such as take deep breaths, or smile and wave to other drivers. Turn the obstacle into an opportunity, and regard the time as a chance for some peace and contemplation instead.

♦ Drive steadily. Accelerate and brake smoothly – don't stamp on the pedals or swerve from one lane to another, it only makes you feel more stressed. How many times have you been overtaken by an impatient driver, only to pull up alongside him at the next set of lights? Speeding doesn't get you there any faster.

168. SIT MORE EFFICIENTLY

The Alexander Technique is popular among musicians, dancers and athletes for creating a more comfortable and efficient posture. According to teachers of the Technique, the root cause of many physical problems is the way we unconsciously and habitually move our bodies. By changing these ingrained habits and functioning in a more efficient, less stressful manner, you can correct postural problems that lead to pain and tension, particularly when you're sitting for long periods.

Practise these positioning tips until they become second nature.

◆ Sit directly on top of your 'sitting bones', and lengthen your torso.

◆ Let your elbows float out and away from your body to widen your shoulders.

◆ Allow your knees to move forward and away from each other so the hip joints move freely.

◆ Use your whole back as a unit, bending from the hip joints rather than always from the waist.

◆ At frequent intervals, get up and walk around the room.

169. SLEEP SOUNDLY

The following exercise, performed while you are lying in bed, is a simple way of calming your mind and muscles before sleep.

◆ Curl up in the foetal position and rock back and forth. This allows you to get in touch with your most primitive feelings so you can feel them, then let them go, and relax.

◆ Now, lie flat on your back with your arms beside you. Take a few deep breaths and imagine all tension leaving your body.

◆ Beginning at your feet, flex and tense them as hard as you can, hold for a few seconds, then relax. Point your toes and tighten your calf muscles. Hold for a few seconds, then relax.

◆ Repeat this process for each set of muscles in your body, working up your legs to your buttocks and lower back. Tighten your back muscles by raising your shoulders up to your ears and then relaxing. Continue the process for your hands, arms and neck.

◆ Finish by pulling a face with your jaw clenched, and then relaxing, and another with your jaw open, and then relaxing.

◆ Breathe deeply, keeping your focus on your breath. Check your body for any residual tension and, if you find any, tighten the area and relax once more. With each exhalation, imagine all remaining tension leaving your body.

'Let food be thy medicine.'

HIPPOCRATES

Nourish . . .

The path to peace of mind and total wellness starts with choosing foods that nourish mind and body, and eating them in a calm fashion. You are what you eat, so if junk goes in, junk comes out; what you eat impacts on your brain function as well as whether you feel sluggish or have plenty of energy.

To stay focused and alert, a certain sense of urgency and an amount of stress and excitement is necessary. Too much, though, and you risk feeling overwhelmed and burned out – just the recipe to fuel cravings for foods high in fat and sugar. Ironically, snacks like a packet of crisps or a chocolate bar only lead to more fatigue and stress. Tension-fuelled food cravings for 'comfort foods' that are high in fat, sugar and salt also make you fat, and play havoc with your metabolism.

All energy enters your body through your food, so the quality of your food plays an enormous role in the energy you bring to the world. Stress promotes a pattern of skipping meals and then overeating, which leads to a roller-coaster ride of energy peaks and troughs, with your emotions, moods and concentration all following your glucose levels. To keep your energy levels balanced and reduce stress, think more about what you should eat, and less about what you shouldn't eat. For example, eating a tryptophan-rich food in the evening such as turkey or peanut butter can significantly improve sleep and regulate mood. Slow-burning foods such as fibre-rich whole grains, vegetables and fruit keep hunger at bay for longer and help balance blood sugar because they are digested more slowly and therefore provide the body with a steadier supply of glucose. Also, it's pointless eating a diet rich in nourishing foods if your body isn't absorbing it correctly, so you need to consider enzyme-rich foods and supplements such as wheatgrass and pawpaw that break down food and allow nutrients to be absorbed by your body.

Aim to eat calmly, simply and cleanly. Chef and restaurateur Neil Perry says, 'Food that is thought about is remembered'. Think about what you are proposing to make or to eat, and create sufficient time to browse for quality food that hasn't been accelerated with growth hormones, genetic manipulation or processing techniques. Avoid rich sauces and fussy trimmings – cook foods simply and lightly. Far from taking more time, selecting basic ingredients of the highest possible quality actually results in tastier, healthier food that is easy to prepare.

Eating less, but eating better, is less likely to lead to weight problems. Wolfing down food doesn't give your body time to signal that you're full. It takes up to 15 minutes for the stomach to send the brain a signal that it's full, so if you eat too quickly, you're almost guaranteed to overeat. Ironically, our bodies evolved when food was scarce and we had to work hard to hunt and gather it. We are actually designed to eat as much as we can as often as we can, storing any excess as fat for burning during times of scarcity. In short, you are genetically programmed to overeat. While you can't change your genetic make-up, being aware of this risk of over-supply and over-demand can help you counter it with simple solutions. For example, doing something other than eat when you're under pressure, or cooking ahead of time so you're not tempted to buy a fatty takeaway when you're pressed for time during the week.

Practising discipline with food also makes for more enjoyable mealtimes, because rather than rushing through your food in a panic, or distracting yourself with a newspaper or the TV while you eat, you learn to savour the sensory qualities of the taste, texture and aroma of your food. Learn to eat mindfully instead of mindlessly. Whether you are at home or in a restaurant, slow down before a meal, no matter how casual or brief, and share a moment of silence at the table or say a few words of gratitude for the food before you eat. Or make an affirmation that you will eat in peace and enjoy your own or other people's company. Eating with gratitude – not only for your body but for your heart and mind as well – may affect how well food is metabolised.

Try to always eat in a relaxed setting. Arrange your table so you have a pleasant view, whether it's of a window or a painting. Choose comfortable chairs. Food nourishes optimally when it is consumed in a peaceful environment, at a calm pace, and with enjoyable company. What you eat is certainly important, but how and with whom you eat is also essential to your physical and mental health. Finally, if you find yourself mindlessly opening the refrigerator or automatically reaching for the sugar, ask yourself 'Is this really nourishing me?' Look at the deeper issues behind these habits.

170. STOCK A HEALTHY PANTRY

Just because you're short on time doesn't mean you can't eat well. Keep healthy staples such as pasta, frozen chicken breasts, bottled low-fat sauces and fresh vegetables that won't deteriorate too quickly (e.g. green capsicum, onions and carrots) on hand. With a well-stocked pantry, you can throw together a tasty and nourishing meal with little or no planning, and minimal preparation time. Select from the following.

♦ **Protein** Milk, soy, beans, fish, eggs and meat all provide sustained energy and help balance blood sugar. Stock up on bean dip, water-packed tuna, fat-free dairy, soy cheese and burgers or sausages, prepared hummus and frozen seafood.

♦ **Carbohydrates** Bread, pasta, cereal, fruits and starchy vegetables supply fuel for your body and brain. Make sure you buy whole-grain varieties. Keep instant porridge, couscous and quick-cook brown rice in your pantry, and buy wheatgerm to sprinkle on cereal or in smoothies.

♦ **Fruits and vegetables** Colourful produce, e.g. leafy greens, oranges, carrots, berries and red capsicum provide fibre and antioxidant nutrients to ward off disease. Brightly coloured fruits such as tomatoes, grapefruit and raspberries have the highest concentrations of vitamin C, which strengthens the immune system and fights infection. Keep supplies of tomato-based sauces and frozen berries if your weekly eating habits are unpredictable. If you haven't the time to squeeze fresh orange juice, at least buy the calcium and vitamin D-fortified varieties to help maintain healthy bones and soothe nerves.

♦ **'Good fats'** The monounsaturated fats found in nuts and olive oil help you absorb fat-soluble vitamins and phytochemicals.

♦ **Tasty toppings and flavourings** Flaxseed meal, garlic, salsa, nuts, raisins, herbs and spices bring extra nutrients and sensory pleasure to your meals. Make sure your salad dressings are low-fat and your soy sauce is low-salt. Lemon juice is an all-purpose meal brightener.

171. MAKE CHOICES THAT HELP YOU COPE

Eating to maintain physical and mental balance when you're under chronic pressure isn't complicated, but you do have to be conscious of your actions.

◆ **Cut caffeine** A cup of coffee is tempting when you're stressed, but caffeine can linger in your system for hours, amping up the stress response and keeping you awake at night. Coffee also contains compounds that reduce iron absorption. Women already consume too little iron to meet their needs, resulting in fatigue and exhaustion, so coffee only worsens the problem. If you can't give it up altogether, have decaffeinated instead, or just one cup first thing in the morning, well before or after a meal.

◆ **Limit alcohol** An occasional glass of wine is relaxing, but three or four will activate the sympathetic nervous system, causing you to sleep less soundly and wake up tired.

◆ **Drink more water** Every time your body starts to get dehydrated, you'll start feeling tired and stressed. By drinking plenty of water, you'll feel less fatigued and agitated. Check your mouth and lips – if they're dry, drink water.

◆ **Eat mild** Too much chilli or other spices can cause indigestion or heartburn. Avoid the flavour enhancer MSG (monosodium glutamate) as it can cause vivid dreaming and restless sleep.

◆ **Cut back on sugar** Sugar shoves extra kilojoules into your body without adding any nutritional value or energy for those kilojoules. You will experience a very quick surge in blood sugar, but then it goes down just as quickly, crashing into deep tiredness and anxiety.

◆ **Limit your salt intake** If you are particularly prone to stress, cut back salt to 1 teaspoon daily to keep your blood pressure from rising. Cut the salt without losing flavour by choosing low-salt soy sauce and unsalted butter.

◆ **Focus on fibre** Fibre-rich beans, fruits, vegetables and whole grains counter stress-induced digestive upsets and constipation.

◆ **Eat regularly** Skip meals and you only compound the depression, anxiety and fatigue brought on by daily hassles and lack of sleep.

172. TRY DIFFERENT THINGS

Shopping for groceries can easily become a monotonous chore, especially if you have teenage sons like I do – our fridge door goes back and forth like a friendly labrador's tail, and we constantly run out of food. Take a little time to consciously open your mind up to different food-purchasing decisions.

◆ **Slow down** Rather than rush through the supermarket and grab the routine items you always buy, slow down and look at everything, and see if you can discover different ways to satisfy your appetite with healthier foods. Pick different fruits and vegetables you haven't tried before. What looks good? Stop and try the samples being offered. Getting coffee? Pick the organic variety instead. Need canned fruit? Check that it's packed in natural juice, not syrup. Stocking up on soft drink? Try fruit-flavoured drinking yoghurt or mineral water flavoured with natural juice.

◆ **Buy a really good vegetarian cookbook** Thousands of research studies show that people who eat diets rich in fruit and vegetables are at a significantly lower risk of most age-related diseases. Fresh produce is the best dietary source of antioxidants, like vitamin C and beta-carotene. These block damage from oxygen fragments known as free radicals that can lead to cancer. Plant-based diets are also as effective as statin medications in lowering cholesterol and the risk of heart disease. Even if you love your meat and have no intention of giving it up, experimenting with different ways to prepare fruit and vegetables will mean you end up eating more of them. Plant-based meals are exciting, delicious and rich with flavour; meatless meals are not boring.

◆ **Plan once, shop once** Sit down for half an hour on a weeknight or on Sunday morning with your favourite cookbook and plan the week's meals. Then shop once, and be done. You won't believe how much time you save when you plan things instead of picking things up every day; the quality and variety of your food choices will also be more balanced.

173. INVEST IN GOOD TOOLS

Having the right utensils and being aware of the pros and cons to your health of different cooking methods will go a long way towards improving the quality of your nutrition, as well as saving you a lot of time. For example, a food processor will bypass time-intensive dicing and mincing, while a hand-held blender will save you endless time with a whisk or fork.

◆ **Don't nuke** Microwave ovens may be quick, but the 'ping-and-peel-off-the-plastic' school of food preparation won't help your health and wellbeing. A study published in the *Journal of the Science of Food and Agriculture* has found that microwaving zapped up to 97 per cent of the flavonoids (antioxidant compounds that reduce the risk of lung cancer and heart disease) in vegetables. Conventional boiling killed 66 per cent, but steaming only caused a flavonoid loss of less than 10 per cent.

◆ **Buy a slow-cooker** Long-cooked, slow-simmered foods have been the hallmark of many cuisines around the world, including soups and stews such as the French cassoulet and the Moroccan tagine. The hours-long cooking process enriches the flavour of the dish in a way that other methods can't match. It also feeds your spirit to be greeted at the door with tantalising fragrances, knowing that you will eat delicious and sustaining food after a hard day.

◆ **Use cast-iron saucepans** Twenty per cent of women in their childbearing years are iron-deficient, according to the *Journal of the American Dietetic Association*. They're not officially anaemic, but the symptoms are the same – fatigue, susceptibility to colds and infection, difficulty concentrating – and they're all worsened by a stressful lifestyle. To pump up the iron content in your diet, buy sturdy cast-iron saucepans. The mineral leaches out of the pot into the food, boosting iron content several-fold, especially in acidic foods such as spaghetti sauce and tomato-based soups.

174. MAKE YOUR OWN STOCK

Good quality, home-made stock is an incredibly nourishing and restorative general tonic for your whole system. Each sip will contain nerve-soothing calcium, magnesium and phosphorus, which have all been leached from the chicken bones.

This nutritious, slow-cooked recipe can hardly be simpler. Slap it all together, go away and do something else for a couple of hours, then freeze in portion-sized batches and use it to kickstart soups and casseroles for months to come.

CHICKEN STOCK

> 1.8 kg (4 lb) chicken, skinned
> 6 shallots, sliced
> 1 bunch parsley, finely chopped
> salt

- ◆ Place the chicken in a large pot with sufficient water to cover.

- ◆ Bring to the boil, then reduce the heat and simmer, covered, for 1½ hours. Skim the scum from the top.

- ◆ Cool and freeze the stock if storing, or make it into chicken soup – a meal – as follows.

- ◆ Remove the chicken from the stock, cool, then pull the meat from the bones. Shred the meat very finely in a food processor, and return to the pot with parsley, shallots and a little salt. Cook for a further 10–15 minutes.

175. EAT SEASONALLY

Thanks to modern transportation, we can purchase fruit and vegetables from all around the world – grapefruit from Israel, cherries from Canada – at all times of the year. While it's convenient, eating with the seasons helps to keep you connected to the richness and bounty of the year.

Eating seasonally is also a natural way of getting what you need nutrient-wise. The fresher the food, the more likely it is to retain different vitamins, minerals and antioxidants. Nutrients are at their highest levels at the peak of ripeness, so eating a piece of fruit or a vegetable when it's out of season may mean some of those nutrients are lost.

Given that we are running out of petroleum and that we will eventually have to rethink how – or even if – we can ship our food all over the place, eating seasonally is also a more realistic practice in the long term. It's a thoughtful way of taking responsibility for our own nourishment, rather than leaving it up to some faceless corporation. You may not be able to grow your own crops or raise animals, but just by forming relationships with local stores and farmers' markets means you're going to get better produce, service and advice. Ask your local fruit market for what's in season and for locally grown produce.

Even the smallest garden or terrace can be home to tomatoes, runner beans and fresh herbs. Besides saving you money, growing just one or two items of fresh produce is a practical way of gaining control over the quality of your food supply. Some of the most nourishing plants that you can grow from seed are also the easiest, e.g. rocket, Asian greens like bok choy, carrots, corn, green beans, herbs, lettuce, capsicum and tomatoes. It also puts you in touch with what is really of value – the earth, the sunshine, the fresh air.

176. CHOOSE ORGANIC

There are far too many chemicals in our bodies, and most of them made their way there from our plates. Even though agricultural and nutrition experts claim that unacceptably high levels of pesticide residues are only found in a very small percentage of foods, concerns remain about the minor – or 'acceptable' – amounts found in pretty much all conventionally farmed produce. The cumulative effects of chemical additives, including pesticides, herbicides and fungicides, are debatable – the fact is, no one really knows what their long-term effects are. Pesticide manufacturers claim that their products pose little risk to consumers and regulatory agency studies emphasise testing with high doses – but they neglect to mention the chronic low-dose exposure that we typically experience.

The differences between organic and conventional farming practices can have a significant effect on your health and that of your environment. Certain conventionally grown fruits and vegetables, e.g. strawberries and peaches, which are usually heavily sprayed, will, on average, expose you to anywhere up to 30 different pesticides. These chemicals are associated with various disorders and diseases, including cancer, of the reproductive, endocrine and immune systems. Pregnant women and children are especially vulnerable, as pesticides have been linked to developmental and behavioural disabilities and impairment.

To play it safe, select organic foods when you can, wash conventional produce thoroughly, and supplement your diet with antioxidant nutrients that help boost immunity and strengthen your body's resistance to toxins. And remember this: companies used to claim that DDT (a classic example of an endocrine-disrupting pesticide) was safe, right up to the day it was banned. So it's best to take a proactive and preventative approach.

177. RISE AND SHINE

Busy people often skip breakfast. They may well be hungry, but they are so focused on the day ahead, they can't tune in to what their body needs before they begin. However, forgoing breakfast is a big mistake, one that sets up problems for the rest of the day. They're usually starving by 11 a.m., overeat at lunch-time, coast till mid-afternoon when their blood sugar crashes and needs sweets or chocolate to keep going. By the time they get home, they're ready to eat the handle off the fridge.

Finding time for a well-balanced breakfast before you head out the door may be one of the morning's most challenging tasks, but it's essential. Your vital organs need slow-burning nutrition first thing to allow for healthy cell turnover. A well-balanced breakfast keeps you alert throughout the day and helps you look and feel healthy.

Even if you can't stomach the thought of breakfast, you need to make eating within an hour of waking a priority. When you skip breakfast and then eat (or overeat) a big mid-morning snack or lunch, it causes a huge increase in blood sugar. Insulin is released and your blood sugar drops. You end up with an almost nonexistent level of productivity and poor concentration; you feel like going to sleep and your brain switches off.

Breakfast is also crucial in maintaining a healthy weight. So is eating calmly – eating breakfast at your computer or while taking calls makes it more difficult to digest your food. Boycott the morning news during breakfast to avoid unnecessary stress as well. If you must, catch the traffic report and the weather, then turn the TV or radio off.

178. SUPPORT YOUR LIVER

Water is essential to balance all the systems of the body and to keep your mind calm. When you're dehydrated, your body finds it more difficult to clear away the internal and external toxins that build up in the body. Start your day with a glass of water to propel your digestive system, especially your liver, into high gear.

Drink a glass of hot water to which you've added the juice of half a lime, a pinch of cayenne pepper and a little honey to cleanse your body. Lime is a detox diet staple, helping to stimulate digestive juices and the release of bile from the liver. It's also an easy vitamin C boost – a quarter of a lime contains 20 mg vitamin C. Cayenne stimulates the secretion of gastric acids in the stomach and raises the metabolic rate. And don't forget to keep drinking throughout the day – about eight 200 ml glasses should be enough, unless you're very active.

179. SMOOTH YOUR WAY TO HEALTH

It's hard to go past a smoothie for a nutritious breakfast that can be made in a flash, but will provide slow-burning energy to take you through to lunchtime.

This blend provides many essential nutrients, such as carbohydrate, protein, vitamin E, B-group vitamins, zinc and magnesium. Yoghurt is a source of bone-strengthening calcium and also provides friendly bacteria that help to boost immunity. Flaxseed is packed with inflammation-fighting essential fatty acids, and apricots are particularly rich in beta-carotene, one of the most important antioxidants, as well as being a useful source of iron, potassium and fibre.

GET UP AND GO

    10 dried apricots
    200 ml (7 fl oz) low-fat milk or soy milk
    1 small banana, peeled and sliced
    pulp of 1 medium-sized passionfruit
    1 tablespoon flaxseed
    1 tablespoon lecithin
    1 teaspoon brewer's yeast
    honey to taste

◆ Put the apricots in a small bowl and cover with boiling water. Set aside for about 5 minutes.

◆ Drain the apricots and combine with all the other ingredients in a blender, processing until smooth. Serve immediately. Substitute the cold milk or soy milk with warmed milk in the colder months, or if you suffer from poor circulation or a sluggish digestive system.

180. GET YOUR OATS

Oats contain a calming substance called venine, which acts as a tonic that keeps a healthy nervous system functioning and also repairs the damage done to the brain when stress hits.

Take the time to make your own nourishing muesli for the next morning. For just a few minutes' effort, you reap the rewards all the next day.

MUESLI

2 tablespoons rolled oats
1 tablespoon currants or raisins
1 tablespoon finely chopped unblanched almonds
1 teaspoon wheatgerm
1 tablespoon chopped dried fruit, e.g. dried apples, banana chips, pawpaw, pears
2 tablespoons finely chopped hazelnuts
200 ml (7 fl oz) low-fat unsweetened yoghurt
½ red apple, grated
½ green apple, grated
1 orange
honey to taste

◆ Place oats, currants or raisins, almonds, wheatgerm, dried fruit and hazelnuts in a bowl with enough water to cover and refrigerate overnight.

◆ Next morning, strain the oat mixture and combine with the yoghurt. Grate both apples, toss with orange juice, and stir through the yoghurt mixture.

◆ Drizzle with honey to serve.

181. SET A RELAXING TABLE

Mealtime settings and rituals reduce stress, improve digestion and nourish your spirit. Here's how to set a more intimate, soothing table.

◆ **Decorate with something natural** Place a bowl of fresh fruit in the middle of the table, or fill a shallow dish with a couple of flowers, or a handful of pinecones, nuts or shells. Tuck a sprig of fresh mint or a twist of ivy into each napkin. Even the smallest vase with a few fresh leaves will have a cheering and settling effect.

◆ **Dim the lights** A darkened room helps bring focus to the table.

◆ **Add a candle** The flickering light creates a soft, calming atmosphere. Choose candles made from beeswax rather than paraffin.

◆ **Use cloth napkins** It's hard to believe the big difference this one little change makes. Apart from being ecologically responsible, they introduce colour and texture to even the most basic setting for one. Buy earth-friendly cloth made from sustainable fibres, such as colourful hemp-blend, cotton and linen.

◆ **Set a sentimental mood** Scour op shops and garage sales for quirky, unusual accessories, such as mismatched cups and glasses in a favourite colour. Remnants of felt, velvet or lace make delightful runners and place mats that you want to smooth and touch with your fingers, adding to the sensory enjoyment of your food. Be creative and find new uses for little-used items. Haul the sherry glasses and egg cups out of storage, for example, pop a rosebud in each, and put next to each person's place.

182. FOCUS ON FOLATE

Elevated levels of the amino acid homocysteine have long been linked to heart disease, and they are worsened by stress and adrenal exhaustion. Keep homocysteine levels in check by consuming lots of folate, found in liver, yeast extract, wheatgerm and green leafy vegetables, especially spinach and parsley.

This light and easy recipe is an exceptionally nourishing dish and it packs an extra stress-busting punch because it's partnered with almonds, which are high in vitamin E, very protective against heart disease, and nerve-soothing calcium.

SPINACH ALMONDINE

> 1 kg (2 lb) fresh English spinach
> olive oil
> 6 cloves garlic, peeled and minced
> 250 ml (8 floz) light chicken stock (see page 218)
> freshly grated parmesan
> 150 g (5 oz) slivered almonds
> pepper and salt to taste
> unsalted butter

♦ Wash and chop the spinach.

♦ Heat some oil in a saucepan, and cook the garlic, stirring frequently, for 2 minutes. Add the spinach, then the stock, and bring to the boil. Reduce the heat, cover and simmer for 3–5 minutes.

♦ Drain the spinach and transfer to a buttered serving dish. Top with parmesan, almonds, salt and pepper, and dot with butter.

♦ Grill until the almonds are slightly golden, about 2 minutes, then serve.

183. COOK YOUR TOMATOES

Lycopene, the red pigment in tomatoes, is a potent antioxidant. It appears to be better absorbed by the body when the tomatoes are cooked, and combined with a bit of fat such as olive oil. The more lycopene you consume, the better your odds for lowering cardiovascular disease and cancer. Vine-ripened tomatoes have more lycopene than tomatoes picked green and allowed to ripen later on.

This quick and easy Italian-style recipe intensifies the flavour of tomatoes and retains their lycopene content.

OVEN-BAKED TOMATOES

    4 medium-sized Roma (plum or egg) tomatoes
    2 cloves garlic, peeled and crushed
    3 tablespoons finely chopped basil
    1 teaspoon each olive oil and balsamic vinegar
    freshly ground black pepper and salt

◆ Preheat the oven to 200°C (400°F). Grease a shallow baking dish.

◆ Mix the garlic, basil, oil, vinegar, salt and pepper to form a paste.

◆ Halve the tomatoes, cutting a thin slice off the sides to make them sit in the baking dish. Spread the tops of the tomatoes with the garlic mixture.

◆ Bake for 20–25 minutes, or until the tomatoes are soft but not falling apart.

◆ Serve warm.

184. GO FISH

Salmon, haddock, tuna, mackerel, herring, sardines and other cold-water fish are rich in healthy fats known as omega-3 fatty acids, which most people don't get enough of. Omega-3s help reduce joint inflammation, improve brain function, lower blood pressure and LDL cholesterol, and reduce your risk of stroke. The more fish you eat, the greater the benefit; experts recommend up to two or three servings a week.

While fish oil supplements may provide some advantages, eating seafood in its whole, natural state will provide nutrients not present in capsules or tablets, such as amino acids. For a healthy dose of omega-3s, your fish should preferably be baked, grilled or poached as in this delicate-tasting recipe, rather than fried.

SALMON IN GREEN TEA

> 1 tablespoon green tea leaves
> boiling water
> olive oil
> 1 tablespoon dry sherry
> 2 shallots, minced
> 2 small salmon fillets

♦ Place the tea leaves in a pot and pour over the boiling water. Steep for 10 minutes and strain.

♦ Heat the oil. Add the shallots and stir-fry for 1–2 minutes. Add the salmon and cook quickly over a high heat for about 1 minute on each side to seal. Pour in the tea and sherry and poach for another 1–2 minutes, or until the salmon is done to your liking.

♦ Remove the salmon with a slotted spoon and keep warm. Bring the liquid to a boil to reduce, then pour over the salmon. Serve immediately on a bed of rice or couscous with steamed asparagus or snowpeas.

185. BE FULL OF BEANS

A few extra servings each week of humble beans or lentils is an easy way to pump up your intake of fibre and iron. Beans and lentils contain phytochemicals that lower blood cholesterol. They also mix well with meat dishes, and because you're eating less meat you're getting a little less saturated fat.

Make up a batch of this quick and easy dhal and freeze in small containers – an ideal stand-by for busy weekdays.

SPICY RED DHAL

> 250 g (8 oz) split red lentils, rinsed
> 2½ cups water
> olive oil
> 2 small brown onions
> 3 cloves garlic, peeled and chopped
> 1 teaspoon minced chilli
> 1 teaspoon each powdered turmeric, cumin, coriander and cardamom
> 200 g (7 oz) chopped tomatoes

◆ Place the lentils and water in a large saucepan and bring to the boil. Reduce the heat, cover, and simmer for 30 minutes, or until tender.

◆ Meanwhile, heat a little oil in another saucepan and gently fry the onions for 10 minutes, or until soft. Add the garlic, chilli, spices and tomatoes and cook over a low heat, stirring frequently, for 10 minutes.

◆ Combine the onion and lentil mixtures, stirring well. Check the seasoning and serve, or cool and freeze.

186. NIBBLE NUTS

While between 70 and 90 per cent of the kilojoules in nuts come from fat, they're mostly the heart-healthy monounsaturated and polyunsaturated types. Walnuts, in particular, are high in protein, fibre, magnesium, vitamin E and potassium. They are also the only nut that contains alpha-linolenic acid, a type of omega-3 fatty acid typically lacking in the Western diet. Low reserves of linolenic acid can result in a range of symptoms, from dry skin to high blood pressure.

Toasting nuts over direct high heat can destroy fragile omega-3 fatty acids, so enjoy them raw, as in this classic recipe, or just lightly heated.

WALDORF SALAD

> 2 red-skinned apples, washed and sliced
> juice of ½ lemon
> 3 sticks celery, chopped
> 1 handful seedless green grapes
> 2 tablespoons walnut halves, chopped
> 1 tablespoon walnut oil

◆ Toss the apple slices in lemon juice to prevent discolouration.

◆ Combine all the ingredients and serve at room temperature.

187. TREAT YOURSELF TO BLUEBERRIES

Blueberries are traditionally enjoyed in the warmer months for their refreshing flavour, but these pretty berries are more than just a summer dessert. Blueberries are a concentrated source of antioxidants that help the body resist infection. A food's antioxidant power is measured in ORAC units (which stands for 'oxygen radical absorbance capacity'), and blueberries rate the highest of any fruit or vegetable. In addition, the pigments that give them their colour support the health of your eyes, and they contain proanthocyanadins (the same sort of tannins that are in cranberries) that help counter the bacteria that cause urinary tract infections.

Keep a couple of packs of frozen berries in your freezer and enjoy this fresh-tasting recipe year-round for its nourishing and immune-enhancing health rewards.

BERRY NICE SOUP

> 500 g (1 lb) mixed berries, e.g. blueberries, raspberries, blackberries, fresh or frozen
> 2 cups water, or a mix of juice from the drained fruit
> 50 ml (¼ cup) apple cider vinegar
> zest of 1 lemon
> juice of 1 orange
> 1 x 5 cm (2 in) cinnamon stick
> a few cloves
> honey to taste
> light sour cream to taste

◆ If using frozen fruit, defrost. If using fresh fruit, pick over the fruit and remove any stalks.

◆ Combine the water or water–juice mix with vinegar, zest, juice, cinnamon and cloves in a large non-aluminium saucepan. Heat gently for 15 minutes. Sieve to remove the spices; discard.

◆ Add the fruit and cook for a further 10 minutes. Purée the mixture in a food processor or blender until smooth. Add honey to taste.

◆ Chill for 2 hours before serving. To serve, swirl in a spoonful of sour cream.

188. EAT MORE ONIONS

Just one inexpensive and flavoursome food can do so much for your health. Onions help reduce total cholesterol and high blood pressure. Quercetin, a flavonoid onions contain, has anti-cancer properties, and fights viral and bacterial infections. Onions are useful in treating asthma because they reduce constriction of the bronchial passageways.

If you're not keen on the volatile smell and strong taste of raw onions, slow cooking is a very mellow way of eating them. This nourishing recipe practically cooks itself with very little effort from you. Make up a batch on a back burner next time you're standing at the stove getting dinner ready, then store it and use on sandwiches, in salads, or as an accompaniment to cold cuts during the week.

Greek Onion Relish

> 250 g (8 oz) white onions, finely chopped
> 2 lemons, sliced and finely chopped
> 3 tablespoons olive oil
> 3 tablespoons dry white wine
> 6 cloves garlic, peeled and minced
> 1 teaspoon peppercorns
> 1 tablespoon pitted Kalamata olives, minced
> 1 tablespoon chopped fresh basil
> 1–2 teaspoons minced chilli

♦ Place onions, lemons, oil, wine, garlic and peppercorns in a small saucepan. Simmer, covered, for 30–45 minutes, stirring occasionally until the mixture is very soft.

♦ Stir through the olives, basil and chilli, adjusting the seasoning if necessary. Serve warm or cold.

189. TAKE THREE CLOVES

If you only do one thing to improve your eating habits each week, add just three cloves of raw garlic to your diet. Garlic is astonishingly good for you, especially if you eat it raw as heat can destroy some of its beneficial properties.

For centuries, garlic has played a major role in medicine, and science continues to confirm its phenomenal health benefits. In particular, garlic protects against heart disease and stimulates your immune system. It also protects against bacterial infections and its sulphur-containing compounds help fight cancers of the skin, stomach, breast and colon. As a natural antioxidant, garlic protects your cells from degenerative changes, especially in the liver and the brain.

Three cloves may sound daunting, but it's very easy, especially if you whip up a batch of this deliciously addictive hummus. Spread it on fresh bread, whisk some into a salad dressing or use as a dip for vegetables.

GARLICKY HUMMUS

    6 cloves garlic, peeled and crushed
    2 tablespoons olive oil
    2–3 tablespoons tahini
    1 tablespoon natural yoghurt
    1–2 tablespoons lemon juice
    250 g (8 oz) canned cooked chickpeas (garbanzos), drained
    salt to taste
    1 teaspoon grated lemon zest
    ½ teaspoon minced fresh chilli

◆ In a blender or food processor, combine the garlic, olive oil, tahini, yoghurt, lemon juice and chickpeas.

◆ Add a little of the reserved chickpea liquid if necessary to reach the desired consistency. Season with salt and stir in the lemon zest and chilli.

◆ Serve at room temperature or chilled, with rice crackers, fresh vegetable sticks or pita pockets.

190. DIP INTO YOGHURT

Yoghurt, kefir and buttermilk contain active cultures of lactobacillus and bifidobacteria, strains of friendly bacteria that may help boost immunity against common infections, increase the absorption of nutrients, reduce the likelihood of stomach ulcers, prevent some skin disorders, and may even cut the risk of colon cancer. There's also evidence that milk protein and its derivatives may have antibacterial and antiviral effects, and yoghurt is a great source of nerve-soothing calcium.

This easy and tasty dip makes a great salad dressing, or a meal in itself. Choose the low- or non-fat version to keep saturated fat to a minimum.

Nutty Yoghurt Dip

> 100 g (3½ oz) mixed nuts, e.g. cashews, walnuts
> 250 g (8 oz) plain Greek yoghurt
> 1 tablespoon freshly grated parmesan
> 2 cloves garlic, peeled and crushed
> ½ teaspoon each chilli powder and paprika
> a dash of lemon juice
> freshly ground pepper and salt

♦ Grind the nuts in a food processor to form a thick meal.

♦ Mix well with yoghurt, parmesan, garlic and spices. Add lemon juice, and salt and pepper to taste. Serve with grilled vegetables or pita bread.

191. LEARN TO LOVE BROCCOLI

Broccoli is a goldmine of nutrients such as folate, beta-carotene and the phytochemical sulphoraphane, which helps block cancer growth. The vitamin K in broccoli also strengthens bones and so lowers your risk of hip fractures later on. If you really dislike the taste, trick your tastebuds by whirling it up with heaps of other nourishing veggies in this satisfying soup.

Hearty Vegetable Soup

olive oil
2 onions, peeled and chopped
2 celery sticks, chopped
4 small yellow squash, diced
¼ small butternut pumpkin, peeled, seeded and cubed
2 carrots, peeled and chopped
2 potatoes, peeled and chopped
1 small head broccoli, stemmed and chopped
200 g (7 oz) corn kernels
2 cups vegetable stock
1–2 bay leaves
375 g (12½ oz) can chopped tomatoes
3 tablespoons tomato paste (optional)
3 tablespoons chopped fresh herbs, e.g. basil, parsley, dill
freshly ground black pepper and salt

- Heat some oil in a large saucepan and fry the onions for 2–3 minutes. Lower the heat and continue to cook the onions until soft.

- Add the vegetables, except the tomatoes, and cook briefly for 1–2 minutes over a low heat. Add the stock and bay leaves, bring to the boil, then reduce the heat and simmer, covered, for 15 minutes, until the vegetables are spoon-tender.

- Add the tomatoes and tomato paste, if using. Continue to cook for a further 10 minutes.

- Stir in the herbs, and blend in batches in a food processor till smooth. Adjust the seasonings, and serve.

192. SAMPLE SOY

Soy foods lower your risk of heart disease by reducing levels of blood cholesterol. The isoflavones in soy are antioxidants that help reduce blood-clot formation. Soy helps improve bone density, and shows promise in cancer prevention. It also tops the list of calming, stabilising foods, being a high-quality protein whose amino acids convert to neurotransmitters in the brain and to muscle energy in the body. If you use soy as a protein source you have the added advantage of minimising fat and cholesterol intake.

Eat moderate amounts of soy milk and tofu, rather than supplements containing concentrated soy isoflavones.

Tofu & Vegetable Stir-fry

2 tablespoons soy sauce	200 g (7 oz) snowpeas, trimmed
2 teaspoons cornflour	100 g (3½ oz) red capsicum strips
1 tablespoon sherry	100 g (3½ oz) yellow capsicum strips
1 tablespoon rice vinegar	
sesame oil	
1 onion, thinly sliced	
2 cloves garlic, peeled and minced	400 g (14 oz) mixed Chinese vegetables, e.g. bean sprouts, corn spears, bok choy
4 cm (1½ in) piece ginger, peeled and sliced	
2 carrots, peeled and cut into matchsticks	200 g (7 oz) firm tofu, cubed
100 g (3½ oz) broccoli florets	100 g (3½ oz) unblanched almonds, slivered

- ◆ Combine the soy sauce, cornflour, sherry and vinegar in a small jug and stir till smooth. Add enough water to make up 150 ml (⅔ cup), stir and set aside.

- ◆ In a large wok, heat some oil then stir-fry onion and garlic for 2–3 minutes. Add the ginger, carrots and broccoli, and cook for 2 minutes. Lastly, add the snowpeas, capsicum and mixed Chinese vegetables and cook for 2 minutes. Pour over half the sauce, stirring steadily.

- ◆ Add the tofu and almonds and stir-fry for a further 30 seconds. Add a little extra sauce, if desired. Adjust the seasoning to taste and serve immediately.

193. GET MORE MAGNESIUM

One thing you can do to help balance your diet and nourish your body is get more magnesium. Most of us don't get anywhere near enough of this important mineral. That's a problem, because magnesium is necessary for every aspect of the body's function. Magnesium deficiency can trigger anxiety, fatigue, migraines, high blood pressure and asthma. Missing out on magnesium wreaks havoc on muscles, causing cramps. You need magnesium to make your muscles relax; it works in conjunction with calcium, which tightens muscles.

Magnesium is a mild sedative and also suppresses the release of stress hormones like adrenalin, so there's reason to think that a shortage can make stress worse. What's more, it's a vicious cycle. The processes that occur during stress – like the speeding up of your heart rate and increased blood pressure – all require magnesium. That makes the shortage worse, which makes you feel more stressed.

Unless you eat very well, and regularly load up on magnesium-rich foods such as whole grains, nuts, seeds, legumes, wheat bran, brewer's yeast, seaweed and leafy greens, chances are your diet won't be providing the amount of magnesium you need. Either consider taking supplements, or boost your magnesium intake throughout the day with one of these magnesium-rich snacks to balance mind and body.

- 1 tablespoon of almond or cashew butter on a sliced banana.

- 1 tablespoon each of wheat bran and brewer's yeast added to your cereal or muesli, or whizzed in a breakfast smoothie.

- Sprinkle a salad with a cup of sunflower seeds.

194. MAKE AN OIL CHANGE

Both saturated fats (animal foods and large quantities of tropical oils such as coconut) and trans fats (a byproduct of hydrogenating liquid oils, found in margarine and many fried and processed foods) can have a negative effect on your health. Some fats, however, can have a positive effect, especially monounsaturated fats (found in olive oil, avocadoes and almonds) and essential fatty acids (flaxseed and fish oils).

Remove unhealthy oils from your pantry and replace them with cold-pressed, chemical-free options. Choosing the right oils makes for better salads, grills and baking – better nourishment all round. Here's what to put in a healthy, well-balanced shopping trolley, and what to avoid.

◆ **Bin-blended vegetable oils** Often extracted with chemicals such as vegetable and animal-derived shortenings and oils high in polyunsaturates, e.g. corn. Better choices are those oils high in heart-healthy monounsaturates and other important nutrients, e.g. oleic acids and omega-3 fatty acids. Use extra-virgin olive oil for dressings; peanut, sesame, sunflower or avocado for high-heat cooking; safflower oil and canola oil for low-heat cooking. (Canola and sunflower crops are sometimes sprayed with chemical pesticides, so check with the manufacturer, or buy organic.)

◆ **Look for oils that have been cold-pressed** If a label does not say this, chances are it's been chemically extracted using petroleum-based solvents. Although the latter method is cheaper, it can mean your oil contains chemical residues.

◆ **Decipher hidden fats** Unhealthy trans fats are found in partially hydrogenated oil, which in turn is found in commercially prepared cakes, biscuits, margarine, snack foods and processed foods.

◆ **Rethink spreads** Use mashed avocado or fruit purées instead of butter for an easy and nutritious way to maintain texture and flavour and cut the fat.

195. EAT MORE CHOCOLATE

As if you needed encouragement! Chocolate has now being hailed as doing wonders for your stressed-out heart, with studies showing that dark chocolate can decrease arterial stiffness in healthy adults. Chocolate also contains phenols – antioxidants similar to those found in red wine – that have been shown to improve vascular wall tone, lower blood pressure and decrease blood-clotting risk.

Strawberry Fondue

> 1 punnet small strawberries
> 100 g (3½ oz) good quality dark chocolate, chopped
> 2 tablespoons light cream
> 1 tablespoon brandy
> a little low-fat milk

◆ Wipe and pick over the strawberries, discarding any that are bruised or wet. Chill in the fridge while you make the sauce.

◆ Fill the base of a double-boiler saucepan with water, and combine the chocolate, cream and brandy in the top half over a very low heat, stirring until smooth, adding a little milk at a time to thin to your desired consistency. Do not overheat or the chocolate will catch and burn.

◆ Pour the chocolate sauce into a warmed dipping bowl, and give each person a portion of strawberries and a small fork to dip the strawberries into the sauce.

196. TAKE RADICAL ACTION

On the whole, human beings are a well-evolved lot. However, we cannot yet make our own vitamin C, and this is a serious design flaw.

If you only take one vitamin supplement, make it vitamin C. You need this powerful antioxidant to detoxify your body, help create collagen for healthy skin and hair, speed up wound healing, reduce inflammation. Vitamin C boosts immunity and helps neutralise damaging free radicals, rogue cells linked with degenerative diseases such as cancer and heart disease.

Although vitamin C is found in plentiful quantities in food – pawpaw, guava, blackcurrants, green capsicum, broccoli, strawberries, kiwifruit, oranges and cabbages, for example – it is easily compromised by a stressful lifestyle. Smoking, the contraceptive pill, drugs such as tetracycline, aspirin and corticosteroids all lower vitamin C levels. It is also easily lost from storage and cooking.

Look for a supplement that contains vitamin C along with other antioxidants, especially vitamin E, selenium, zinc and beta-carotene or mixed carotenes (including lycopene). Beta-carotene and zinc are vital for maintaining strong immune function, and coenzyme Q10 provides energy to keep you going. Studies show that selenium cuts the risk of lung, colorectal and prostate cancers, and lycopene improves mental agility.

Other safer, smarter alternatives to prescription antidepressants include the B-complex vitamins (for nerve health), the amino acid tryptophan (promotes relaxation), and chromium (for blood sugar imbalances, which cause mood swings, jitteriness and exhaustion).

197. SNACK SMARTER

When you're under pressure, forget the three-meals-a-day routine and eat small, frequent meals and healthy snacks that boost your immune system, balance hormones and nerve chemicals, keep your energy levels up, and your stress levels low. Eating small portions of healthy food about every 3–4 hours allows you to be more flexible without going into overeating mode when you're stressed. These ideas will help keep your blood sugar levels steady and thwart your urge to overeat junk foods, even on your most hectic day. Best of all, they take just seconds to prepare.

- **Banana colada** Whiz together ½ cup plain, low-fat yoghurt, 1 sliced banana, ½ cup pineapple chunks, 3 tablespoons skim milk, 1 tablespoon shredded coconut and a dash of vanilla extract. Bananas contain <u>norepinephrine</u> and serotonin, two brain chemicals that make you calmer and happier.

- **Citrus sparkle** Sprinkle crystallised ginger over vitamin C-rich mandarin slices. Serve with a dollop of lemon yoghurt. Stress depletes your body's supply of vitamin C, and a low supply of vitamin C further raises cortisol levels, aggravating the stress response.

- **Sweet treat** Stuff almonds into dates. Almonds contain magnesium, which is important for maintaining normal sleep patterns.

- **Mini pizza** Toast a wholewheat muffin, top with pizza sauce, sliced veggies and low-fat cheese. Grill for 1 minute, or until the cheese bubbles.

- **Do-it-yourself trail mix** Combine 1 cup mixed nuts (e.g. unsalted cashews, peanuts, walnuts, hazelnuts, pumpkin seeds), 1 cup mixed dried unsulphured fruit (raisins, currants, diced dried apricot and pineapple) plus ½ cup chocolate-coated soy nuts and a shake of cinnamon. Store in an airtight container.

- **Lime-fresh guacamole** Mash together in a bowl ½ cup cubed ripe avocado, 2 tablespoons canned white beans, 2 cloves garlic, 1 teaspoon lime juice and ½ teaspoon ground cumin. Serve with half a toasted wholewheat pita pocket, cut into wedges.

198. SWAP, DON'T DROP

It is much easier to substitute products and ingredients than to try and drop ingrained eating habits altogether. Some examples:

- **Miso *v*. morning coffee** Made from fermented soybeans, miso is a nourishing protein-rich beverage that takes only seconds to prepare. Snip open a sachet, squeeze the contents into a cup and pour boiling water over. Inhale the rich, savoury aroma and take a moment to reclaim your scattered thoughts.

- **Alfalfa instead of iceberg** No wonder cows look so contented munching away – they're often chewing on alfalfa, which is naturally high in nerve-soothing minerals and has an alkalinising effect on the digestive system. Use on sandwiches and in salads rather than nutrient-poor lettuce.

- **Add** a shot Wheatgrass packs a punch nutrition-wise, providing a bumper dose of vitamin C and chlorophyll to detoxify the body, as well as a long list of trace elements. Buy or make a sprouter (see page 23) and grow your own wheatgrass on a kitchen windowsill so you can add it to your morning juice. Or buy the pre-packaged shots and just snip and stir.

- **Sprinkle seeds** Instead of shaking a spoonful of sugar over morning cereal or adding salt to soups or casseroles, make this tasty, nutty alternative. Mix together roughly equal amounts of the following: flax, sunflower, pumpkin and sesame seeds, and wheatgerm. Grind them well, using a herb or coffee grinder, then store in an airtight container in the fridge for up to 5 days. Seeds are a rich source of essential fatty acids, which play a powerful role in countering stress responses. They also moderate the body's production of natural inflammatory substances, which in turn encourage the release of too much cortisol. Wheatgerm is the heart of the wheat kernel, and is a goldmine of nutrition, providing generous amounts of magnesium as well as folate and vitamin E. Wheatgerm also provides respectable amounts of trace minerals often missing in the modern diet, especially zinc.

◆ **Pick edamame, not crisps** Fun to say (eh-dah-mah-may) and fun to eat, these bright-green young soybeans, which look similar to sugar snap peas, have an addictively sweet and nutty flavour. They are sold shelled or in their pods at farmers' markets, Asian food stores and some supermarkets. They make terrific garnishes for soups, salads and rice dishes, and are a delightful snack as well as an easy way of boosting your daily vegetable intake.

◆ **Trade in your regular potatoes for sweet potatoes** They outshine the ordinary spud when it comes to providing vitamins and minerals, including more than six times the amount of bone-building calcium and a generous quantity of beta-carotene, which lowers the risk of heart disease and cancer.

◆ **Sweeten with honey, not sugar** As well as being a great source of energy, the darker the honey, the more nerve-soothing trace minerals and vitamins it provides. Add to hot and cold drinks, or spread on a wholewheat muffin for a quick, nourishing snack.

◆ **Swap refined grains** like white rice for fibre-rich whole grains and wheat alternatives, e.g. quinoa and millet. Whole grains are far superior nutritionally to refined varieties because they retain the germ – rich in heart-supporting vitamin E – and folate, and the bran, a source of fibre. Fibre lowers cholesterol, prevents constipation, slows digestion to help steady blood sugar levels, and makes you feel fuller faster, which curbs overeating and weight gain. Whole grains also win hands down when it comes to providing more nutrients, including nerve-soothing B-group vitamins, copper, chromium, zinc and magnesium.

◆ **Go for bold, not bland** Make sure each plateful of food contains at least three colours. Many nutrients manifest themselves as colour, so you're making certain that the meal looks appealing and appetising as well as ensuring that you have a healthy variety of food.

199. TURN OVER A NEW LEAF

When George Orwell wrote, 'A perfectly made cup of tea brings the sipper nothing less than wisdom, bravery, and renewed optimism', he tapped into the heart of a stress-reducing tradition that has stood the test of time for good reason. Throughout the ages, almost every culture in the world has used plants for healing and to help calm the mind and relax the body. The study of plants and their therapeutic uses continues, with scientific research regularly confirming that many herbs are effective in reducing stress.

Slowing down and finding balance in your life can be as simple as preparing a hot cup of herbal tea. There's a special kind of magic to be found in tea-making, as the elemental forces of fire, water and earth come together. You concoct a recipe of roots and leaves, flowers and seeds, add boiling water, and watch your potent brew steam and simmer. The ritual of making tea, letting it steep and breathing in the soothing, head-clearing scent, then closing your eyes as you sip is a healing and balancing act, appeasing all five senses, and creating harmony. Feel the warm steam play over your tired eyelids and imagine it clearing your mind.

In nature, plants – like people – are happiest when they can live and grow together, rather than alone. They also work better as medicine when taken synergistically, and they taste better when taken together, when the flavours support and enhance each other. Blending your own herb tea is an easy and satisfying way to reconnect with nature and restore your body and spirit. Blends are simple and safe; the herbs themselves are versatile and readily available from good healthfood stores. Try these following combinations. Use 1–2 teaspoons of your blend per cup of boiling water, and steep for 10 minutes.

- **Peppermint and chamomile** Both herbs are excellent for the relief of tension headaches and digestive problems brought on by nervous upsets. This is also a relaxing drink before bed. Add the strained tea to a hot bath to help relax muscles and reduce fatigue.

- **Lavender and orange peel** Lavender is a gentle sedative. Orange peel adds a delicate, warming flavour and its scent boosts mood and motivation, while being warming and comforting at the same time. Try this tea if you are anxious or have difficulty sleeping.

♦ **Lemon balm and passionflower** The seventeenth-century herbalist Nicolas Culpeper wrote that 'lemon balm driveth away all melancholy', and science does, in fact, indicate that lemon balm is exceptionally tranquillising. This herb has been used in aged care units to calm agitated patients, and to reduce their reliance on pharmaceutical relaxants and sedatives. Passionflower is calming, helps promote sleep and helps relieve cramping and indigestion. Drink this tea to decompress after a tough day.

Make your tea-making ritual an oasis of calm in your day. Collect and set aside exquisite accoutrements – a special silver spoon, a pretty tea ball, elegant bone china cups or mugs, and golden honey – and choose organically grown herbs for total sensory gratification. More than that, they will enrich your health and exalt your spirit.

ACKNOWLEDGEMENTS

Thank you to my publisher Sue Hines, my in-house editor Andrea McNamara, my agent Margaret Connolly and copyeditor Foong Ling Kong. Thanks also to Jennifer Castles, publisher's assistant at A&U and Slow Up cover model, and to photographer Monty Coles and designer Nada Backovic for creating such an inspiring design for this book.

INDEXES